ABC of

Common Soft Tissue Disorders

EDITED BY

Francis Morris

Consultant in Emergency Medicine
Northern General Hospital
Sheffield
UK

Jim Wardrope

Emeritus Consultant in Emergency Medicine
Northern General Hospital
Sheffield
UK

Paul Hattam

Principal Physiotherapist and Director
The Physios
Sheffield
UK

WILEY Blackwell

BMJ|Books

Library of Congress Cataloging-in-Publication Data

Names: Morris, Francis, editor. | Wardrope, Jim, editor. | Hattam, Paul, editor.
Title: ABC of common soft tissue disorders / edited by Francis Morris, Jim Wardrope, Paul Hattam.
Other titles: ABC series (Malden, Mass.)
Description: Chichester, West Sussex, UK ; Hoboken, NJ : John Wiley & Sons Inc., 2016. | Series: ABC series | Includes bibliographical references and index.
Identifiers: LCCN 2015047748| ISBN 9781118799789 (pbk.) | ISBN 9781118799765 (Adobe PDF) | ISBN 9781118799772 (ePub)
Subjects: | MESH: Soft Tissue Injuries–diagnosis | Soft Tissue Injuries–therapy | Musculoskeletal Pain–diagnosis | Musculoskeletal Pain–therapy
Classification: LCC RC925.5 | NLM WO 700 | DDC 616.7–dc23 LC record available at http://lccn.loc.gov/2015047748

A catalogue record for this book is available from the British Library.

Wiley also publishes its books in a variety of electronic formats. Some content that appears in print may not be available in electronic books.

Cover image: ©Halfpoint/Getty images

Typeset in 9.25/12pt MinionPro by SPi Global, Chennai, India
Printed and bound in Singapore by Markono Print Media Pte Ltd

1 2016

ABC of
Common Soft Tissue Disorders

WITHDRAWN

ABC series

An outstanding collection of resources for everyone in primary care

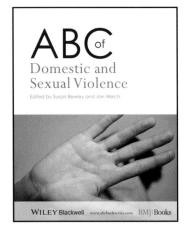

ABC of Domestic and Sexual Violence

Edited by Susan Bewley and Jan Welch

WILEY Blackwell www.abcbookseries.com BMJ|Books

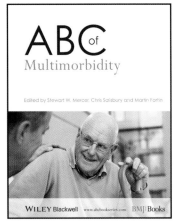

ABC of Multimorbidity

Edited by Stewart W. Mercer, Chris Salisbury and Martin Fortin

WILEY Blackwell www.abcbookseries.com BMJ|Books

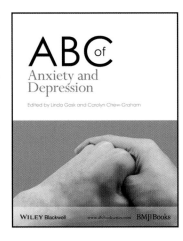

ABC of Anxiety and Depression

Edited by Linda Gask and Carolyn Chew-Graham

WILEY Blackwell www.abcbookseries.com BMJ|Books

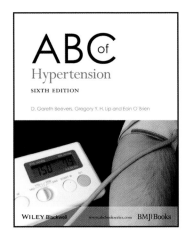

ABC of Hypertension

SIXTH EDITION

D. Gareth Beevers, Gregory Y. H. Lip and Eoin O'Brien

WILEY Blackwell www.abcbookseries.com BMJ|Books

The *ABC* Series contains a wealth of indispensable resources for GPs, GP registrars, junior doctors, and all those in primary care

- **Highly illustrated, informative, and practical**

- **Covers the symptoms, investigations, and treatment and management of conditions presenting in daily practice**

- **Full colour photographs and illustrations aid diagnosis and patient understanding**

For more information on all books in the ABC series, including links to further information, references and links to the latest official guidelines, please visit:

www.abcbookseries.com

BMJ|Books

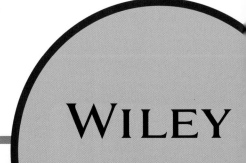

WILEY

Contents

List of Contributors

Rahul Anaspure, MBBS, MRCS, FRCR
Consultant Musculoskeletal Radiologist, Royal Devon & Exeter Hospital, Exeter, UK

Michael Athanassacopoulos, MD
Consultant Spinal Surgeon, Sheffield Teaching Hospitals NHS Foundation Trust, Sheffield, UK

Chris M. Blundell, BMedSci (Hons), MBChB, MD, FRCS (Tr & Orth)
Claremont Private Hospital, Sheffield, UK

Carolyn Chadwick, FRCS Ed (Tr & Orth)
Consultant Orthopaedic Surgeon, Sheffield Teaching Hospitals NHS Foundation Trust, Sheffield, UK

Neil Chiverton, FRCS Ed (Tr & Orth)
Consultant Spinal Surgeon, Sheffield Teaching Hospitals NHS Foundation Trust, Sheffield, UK

Ben Cooper, MBChB, FCEM
Consultant in Emergency Medicine, Sheffield Teaching Hospitals NHS Foundation Trust, Sheffield, UK

Helen Cugnoni, FRCP, FRCS, FCEM
Consultant in Emergency Medicine, Homerton University Hospital, London, UK

Roger Dalton, MB, ChB, FRCEM
EM Consultant and Sports Physician, Chesterfield FC, Chesterfield, UK

Mark B. Davies BM, FRCS (Tr & Orth)
Consultant Orthopaedic Foot and Ankle Surgeon, Sheffield Teaching Hospitals NHS Foundation Trust, Sheffield, UK

Richard J. Follett, BSc, MCSP, HPC
Physiotherapist, Director, Fit4-Physio, Sheffield, UK

Lennard Funk, BSc, MSc, FRCS (Tr & Orth), FFSEM(UK)
Consultant Shoulder Surgeon and Professor of Orthopaedics and Sports Science, Wrightington, Wigan & Leigh NHS Trust, Wrightington, UK

Sherif Hemaya, MBChB, FCEM
Consultant in Emergency Medicine, Sheffield Teaching Hospitals NHS Foundation Trust, Sheffield, UK

Ashley Jones, BSc (Sports Therapist)
Sports Therapist, Chesterfield FC, Chesterfield, UK

David Knott, MB, BS
Clinical Lead, Orthopaedic Practitioner, Dorset HealthCare University NHS Foundation Trust, Poole, UK

Joanna Ollerenshaw, BSc (Hons), MSc, MCSP, SRP
Extended Scope Practitioner Physiotherapist, Sheffield Teaching Hospitals NHS Foundation Trust, Sheffield, UK

Hasan Qayyum, FRCEM
Consultant in Emergency Medicine, Sheffield Teaching Hospitals NHS Foundation Trust, Sheffield, UK

Alison Smeatham, MSc, MCSP, FSOM
Extended Scope Practitioner, Royal Devon & Exeter Hospital, Exeter, UK

David Stanley, FRCS (Tr & Orth)
Consultant in Orthopaedics, Shoulder and Elbow Unit, Northern General Hospital, Sheffield Teaching Hospitals NHS Foundation Trust, Sheffield, UK

Paul M. Sutton, MBChB, FRCS (Tr & Orth)
Sheffield Orthopaedics Ltd, Sheffield, UK

Santosh Venkatachalam, FRCS (Tr& Orth)
Consultant in Orthopaedics, Northumbria Healthcare, North Tyneside General Hospital, North Shields, UK

Jim Wardrope, MBChB, FRCS, FRCEM, CBE
Emeritus Consultant in Emergency Medicine, Northern General Hospital, Sheffield, UK

CHAPTER 1

Introduction to Musculoskeletal Medicine

Jim Wardrope

Northern General Hospital, Sheffield, UK

OVERVIEW

- This chapter will review the structure of the musculoskeletal system and how the 'human machine' works.
- How the musculoskeletal system is modified by age and illness.
- A *system* is outlined for history, examination, investigations and note taking.
- The principles of management of injury to muscles, tendons, ligaments and nerves are examined.
- How best to restore function is discussed.

Introduction

Musculoskeletal conditions are one of the commonest presentations in general practice. One in four people at any one time will have a musculoskeletal problem. Such conditions are responsible for one in seven primary care consultations. Almost 50% of the population will have back pain in 1 year. The cost to society is huge.

These conditions are often regarded by doctors as 'minor' problems, but to patients they are often painful and disabling. Very occasionally apparently minor problems can be life threatening.

Structure and function: the body as a machine

The skeleton

Any machine needs a rigid framework. The main functions of this framework are to overcome the effects of gravity, to protect vital parts and to provide a network of levers to enable the effective application of force.

A crane shows these functions as well (Figure 1.1). It has a network of steel girders to give it height (overcome gravity) and a very long arm to provide a means of reaching and for the effective application of force. It has specialized areas for protection, for example the driver's cab (skull). The human skeleton is much more complex but the principles are the same. The 'girders' of the skeleton are the bones, designed by evolution to be strong, to have some elasticity but still to be light.

Joints

The crane has a few simple joints that allow movement, flexibility and a degree of shock absorption. At the base there is a circular joint to allow 360° motility in one plane. It comprises load-bearing surfaces, lubrication and constraining structures that hold the joint in place. The nearest human equivalent would be a ball-and-socket joint such as the shoulder. There are also hinge-type joints allowing motion in one plane (e.g. the elbow).

Human joints are much more complex and of greater variety (synovial, symphyseal and syndesmotic). These joints all have articular surfaces, and ligaments that connect the bones together, and also contain stretch receptors and associated muscles. They may also have specialized structures such as intra-articular cartilages that may assist in shock absorption or in joint stability.

Muscles and tendons

The powerhouse needs a fuel supply, oxygen, a method of converting the energy in the fuel to mechanical energy and a method of transmission of that energy to the skeleton. Skeletal muscle uses sugar as its main energy source backed up by glycogen to meet the peak action of the 'pistons' of the actin and myosin filaments that cause contraction (and relaxation).

The muscle exerts its force through tendons. Tendons are immensely strong yet also have elastic stretch. This stops them breaking at times of sudden loading (see Figure 1.2).

Reciprocal groups of muscles

An important concept is that with many active muscle movements there are opposing muscles which contract to allow a stable platform for the active muscle. Using the crane analogy, the large counterbalance weight is essential to prevent the crane toppling over when lifting a load (see Figure 1.1). A good example of this is tennis elbow. There is pain at the extensor origin when gripping. The main active muscles are the finger flexors; however, the extensors of the wrist have to contract to stabilize the wrist. Without this reciprocal action the wrist would flex and grip strength would be lost. This powerful

ABC of Common Soft Tissue Disorders, First Edition.
Edited by Francis Morris, Jim Wardrope and Paul Hattam.
© 2016 John Wiley & Sons, Ltd. Published 2016 by John Wiley & Sons, Ltd.

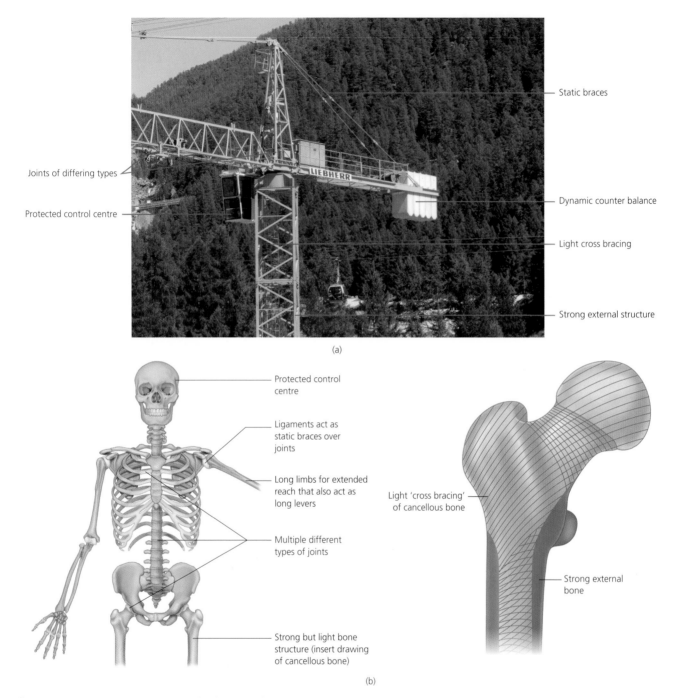

Static braces

Dynamic counter balance

Light cross bracing

Strong external structure

Joints of differing types

Protected control centre

(a)

Protected control centre

Ligaments act as static braces over joints

Long limbs for extended reach that also act as long levers

Multiple different types of joints

Strong but light bone structure (insert drawing of cancellous bone)

Light 'cross bracing' of cancellous bone

Strong external bone

(b)

Figure 1.1 A crane is a very simple machine but has many elements in common with the human body. The human body is subject to the laws of mechanics like any other machine.

reciprocal contraction causes stress at the origin of the wrist extensors at the lateral epicondyle (see Figure 1.3).

Nerves

All machines need a control system. The brain, the spinal cord and the motor and sensory nerves provide that control system.

Much of the control of movement is carried on at an unconscious level. The simplest example of unconscious control is the spinal stretch reflex. If a muscle is stretched, then receptors in the muscle and tendon are activated, and signals are passed up the sensory nerves to the spinal cord and hence to the motor neurones that fire to cause the reflex contraction. This reflex arc is subject to many other influences, both from within the spinal cord and descending from the cerebellum and the cerebral cortex and associated nuclei. However, it is a key concept in understanding the importance of muscle power and the neural control in maintaining joint stability (see below).

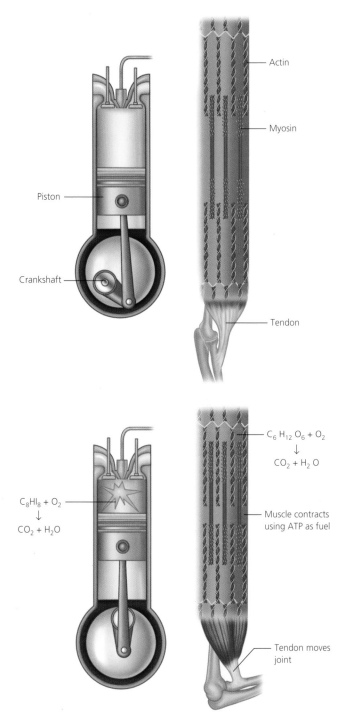

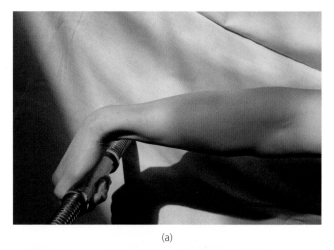

(a)

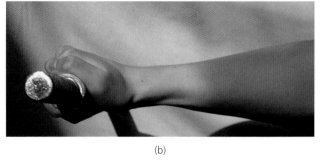

(b)

Figure 1.3 Reciprocal muscle contraction. In gripping the finger flexor muscles contact strongly. If the wrist extensors do not 'brace' the wrist then the wrist would also flex and grip would be very weak (a). Strong contraction of the wrist extensors allows the finger flexors to exert maximum power (b).

Figure 1.2 The human 'combustion engine'. (a) Fuel in a car engine is combusted with oxygen to create a force that moves the piston and turns the crankshaft. (b) Glucose in muscle cells is respired to create the ATP that drives muscle contraction.

Functions and stresses

The human body is a complex system of levers. In clinical practice we tend not to think of the physics of movement and function but understanding the rudiments of biomechanics is key to the practice of musculoskeletal medicine. We can only skim the surface of this subject but further information can be found in *The human machine* (McNeill 1992) or *Physics in biology and medicine* (Davidovits 2008).

Take the example of lifting a simple weight. If incorrect lifting technique is used, then the spine becomes a very long arm of a lever that has to support not only the weight being lifted but the weight of the upper body (Figure 1.4). The fulcrum of this lever is the lumbosacral junction. The forces across this joint are huge: lifting a 10 kg weight with an extended spine results in 0.5 tonne of force.

If the forces are so huge, why do we not fall apart? The musculoskeletal system has many modifications that allow it to withstand these forces. Many of the structures are immensely strong yet have a certain degree of elasticity that prevent failure with sudden peak loading. However, it is the 'dynamic stability' of muscle power that provides the majority of joint stability. For example:

- ankle is inverted,
- stretch receptors in the ligaments, evertor tendons and muscles are activated,
- a reflex contraction of the evertor muscles corrects the deforming force,
- ankle stability is protected (see Figure 1.5).

This contraction can be so strong that it may pull off the evertor attachment (fracture of the fifth metatarsal styloid process) or the tendon may snap.

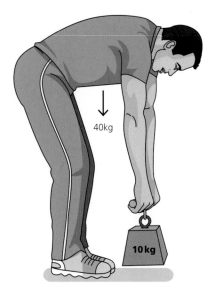

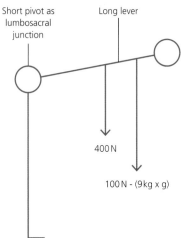

Figure 1.4 Lifting a 10 kg weight the wrong way, with a bent back. Upper body weight is 40 kg. The resultant force is weight in kg × acceleration of gravity: $(40\,kg + 10\,kg) \times 10\,m/s^2 = 500\,N$. This force is acting over a 1 m lever (distance between the fulcrum at the lumbosacral joint and the shoulders), giving a resulting moment of 500 Nm. The opposing lever at the lumbosacral joint is much shorter, approximately 10 cm. The moment that needs to be generated over this short 10 cm lever is 500 Nm, thus requiring 5000 N of force over the lumbosacral joint.

If a joint is immobilized then two things happen: the speed of the stretch reflex is delayed and muscle bulk and power are lost. This is a key concept that demonstrates the absolutely vital importance of rehabilitation in the management of many musculoskeletal injuries. A simple grade 1 ankle sprain can result in wasted calf muscles and an unstable ankle if immobilization or non-weight bearing is prolonged.

Effects of age, other morbidity, drugs and training

Unlike machines the human body does not come to an exact specification. While it is true that machines will age and the various parts will become prone to failure, they are not subject to the huge variation in that is seen in the population attending the clinic or surgery.

As the population ages the burden of illness in the community rises exponentially. Age-related changes affect the structure and functioning of the musculoskeletal system.

- The skeleton becomes more brittle, resulting in an increase in fractures, often with little or no trauma.
- Muscle bulk is lost, resulting in a loss of capacity to withstand stresses across joints.
- Reflexes slow, resulting in less stability as a whole and a higher incidence of falls.
- Tendons lose strength, resulting in more tendon ruptures such as quadriceps tendon.
- Diabetes now affects 2% of the population. These patients are at very significantly increased risk of infections and vascular disease. The early stages of severe foot infections or peripheral vascular disease (PVD) can often present as a musculoskeletal problem. Always take extra care in the assessment of patients with diabetes.
- Anticoagulant drugs, for example warfarin, can result in significant bleeding complications such as muscle haematomas.
- Children have a number of specific types of problem not seen in adults, such as slipped epiphysis, and greenstick and epiphyseal fractures.

Effects of weight

In an 80 kg individual the upper body weight is estimated to be 40 kg. In a 160 kg person with an estimated upper body weight of 80 kg the forces across the lumbosacral junction increase markedly. Another example is the patellofemoral joint. In climbing stairs the quadriceps acts by pushing the patella back against the lower end of the femur (Figure 1.6). The mechanics of this action suggest that the force on the joint is three times the body weight: for a 70 kg individual this is a 2100 N force and for a 150 kg individual it is a 4500 N force. A heavier, fit individual who has stronger structures, stronger muscles and faster reflexes will be able to resist these forces, but if the weight is due to inert fat in an inert individual the chances of injury will be much increased.

Structured assessment

Structured clinical assessment is basic building block of musculoskeletal medicine. A good history and methodical examination are the standard of care expected in this discipline. You may already have a system that works but it should cover the elements set out below. If you use the same system to write up your notes, it acts as a checklist (see Table 1.1). In the complex and busy world of clinical medicine such checklists help reduce error. Pilots use this method and they work with relatively straightforward machines that are all built to the same specification and which are serviced regularly, and they have detailed information about each part of the aeroplane. We work with machines (humans) that come in all shapes and sizes, and many are not well cared for and have parts that are not in proper working order; hence there is even more need for a structured approach.

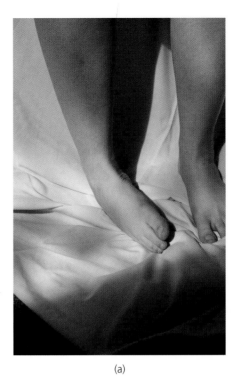
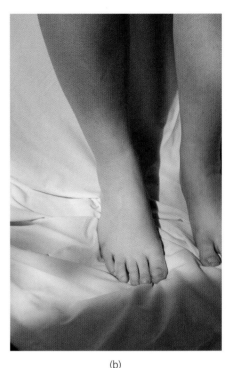

(a)   (b)

Figure 1.5 The ankle inverts, stretch receptors activate (a), there is a reflex contraction of the evertor muscles, the deforming force is overcome and the ankle returns to the normal position (b).

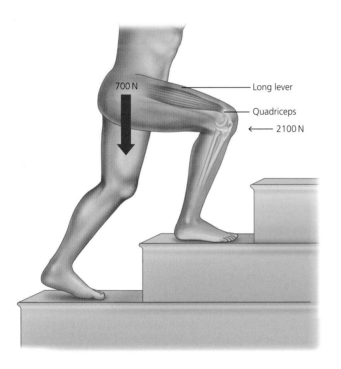

Figure 1.6 In climbing stairs the forces acting on the patellofemoral joint are three times the body weight.

Table 1.1 Musculoskeletal assessment checklist.

History	
Mechanism of injury: trauma versus non-trauma	✓
Symptoms and progress of the symptoms	✓
Previous injury/problems	✓
Past medical history including drugs and allergy	✓
Occupation, sport and hobbies	✓
Examination	
General exam	✓
Limb problems	✓
Function	✓
Joints above and below	✓
Look	✓
Feel	✓
Movement (active/passive/resisted/stress/special tests)	✓
Nerves and vessels	✓

Forces have magnitude, direction and duration. In most injuries the time element is hard to quantify, except in repeated minor forces causing overuse and stress injuries. Having a clear idea of the size and direction of the forces applied gives you a head start in reaching an accurate diagnosis.

Where there is no real history of an injury, the clinician needs to explore the onset and progress of symptoms in great detail, including other symptoms, past medical history and drug history.

Mechanism of injury: trauma versus non-trauma

There is a great difference in the diagnostic spectrum (Table 1.2) between traumatic injuries and non-traumatic musculoskeletal problems. An injury is caused by a force, commonly a single episode of abnormal loading of part of the musculoskeletal system.

Symptoms and progress of the symptoms

Serious injuries usually result in immediate loss of function with significant signs. A good example of this is an acute knee injury (e.g. 'getting carried off' during a football match), with a knee that has swollen immediately. This is a good sign that a serious

Table 1.2 Spectrum of injury in non-traumatic musculoskeletal problems.

Red conditions	Yellow conditions	Green conditions
Potentially life-/limb-threatening: very time-sensitive for treatment	*Potentially limb-threatening/ disabling: may be time-sensitive for treatment*	*Chronic conditions: may be disabling but no time-sensitive element to treatment*
Referred pain	Inflammatory arthropathy	Osteoarthritis
Ischaemia/thromboembolic disease	Crystal arthropathy	Tendonitis
Sepsis	Nerve root/nerve compression	Mechanical back pain
Childrens' problems (e.g. slipped upper femoral epiphysis)	Tumour (primary, secondary, non-metastatic)	
Spinal compression	Stress fractures/tendon ruptures	
	Polymyalgia rheumatica	

intra-articular injury has occurred. In contrast, 'getting a knock' (also during team sport), continuing to play and presenting 2–3 days later with a limp and mildly swollen knee often allows a more leisurely approach to diagnosis.

Ask what treatments have been tried and how these have affected symptoms.

Previous injury/problems

The approach to a single episode of trauma will be different to that for repeated injuries to one part of the body. A single episode of 'I went over on my ankle' is different to 'I keep going over on my ankle'. Patients with repeated problems often require more investigation and treatment.

Past medical history including drugs and allergy

It is always best to ask these questions. Giving a non-steroidal anti-inflammatory drug to a patient with a history of peptic ulcers is contraindicated. Warfarin can turn a minor injury into a major problem because of joint or muscle bleeding.

Occupation, sport and hobbies

Would you treat a knee injury in a professional football player differently from the same problem in a patient with a sedentary job and no active hobbies? Some may say no, but realistically we all would have a different approach. The footballer needs 100% knee function but the person with no active demands may cope well with 80% function or less. Appreciation of the expectations of the patient and the effects of a less-than-perfect recovery are an important dimension to your assessment and treatment plan.

Examination

General exam

Where there is a specific mechanism of injury a general examination is usually not required unless the patient looks unwell, the history is inconsistent or there is a suspicion that the injury was not a straightforward 'mechanical' event (e.g. a dizzy episode, a faint or fit, or non-accidental).

If there is no specific history of injury note the general state of the patient and record at least temperature and pulse. Depending on the clinical situation a more detailed general medical exam, including blood pressure and examination of the major body systems, may be needed, for example in a patient with an injury after a collapse.

Limb problems

Consider the following aspects: function, joints above and below, look, feel, movement (active/passive/resisted/stress/special tests) and nerves and vessels.

- Function: it is usually easy to note if the patient is weight bearing, holding a limb in an awkward way or not using a limb. This can be especially important in children.
- Joints above and below: it is best to screen the rest of the limb for injury. Pain can be referred, the classic error being not to examine the hip in a patient presenting with knee pain. Some injury patterns involve more than one joint (e.g. Maisonneuve injury).
- Look: always compare limbs. Subtle swelling or deformity may be missed if comparison is omitted. Look for swelling, bruising, erythema and deformity (Figure 1.7a).
- Feel: use a single palpating digit to define exact points of tenderness (Figure 1.7b).
- Movement: different types of movement test different structures and can lead to a more accurate diagnosis. Active and passive ranges of movement mostly involve joint function (although pain on passive stretching of a muscle is sign of muscle of muscle or tendon problems (Figure 1.7c). Resisted movement is where the joint is not moving but the muscle, its attachments and tendons are being tested (Figure 1.7d). Stress testing (gentle!) applies force to a joint to check for ligament laxity (Figure 1.7e). There are many special tests that have to be done in certain given clinical presentations; for example, the calf squeeze (Simmond's) test in a patient with sudden onset of pain behind the heel (Figure 1.7f). Such tests may be diagnostic of the injury and failure to perform them might lead to significant errors in management.
- Nerves and vessels: neurovascular exam should be a routine part of the limb examination.

Indications for investigations

We now have the ability to define injuries with a much greater degree of accuracy than before. Ultrasound and magnetic resonance

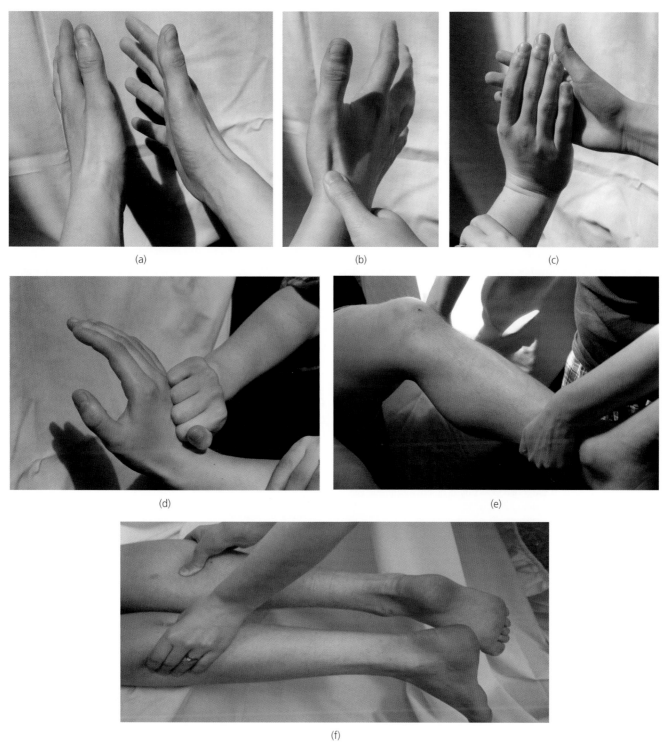

Figure 1.7 (a) Look: always compare sides. (b) Feel: use a single palpating digit to localize tenderness accurately. (c) Active and passive range indicates joint function. (d) Resisted movement indicates muscle/tendon/insertion function. (e) Stress tests indicate ligament function. (f) Special tests may be the only way of making a clinical diagnosis in some conditions.

(MR) scanning have revolutionized the investigation of soft tissue problems. Musculoskeletal problems are so common that to scan everyone would result in vastly increased costs and very long delays in management. Some degree of triage and selection of cases for investigation are needed.

X-rays

In patients with an injury it is often necessary to obtain x-rays to exclude a bony injury. Fortunately there are good-evidence based guidelines to assist the decision, for example the Canadian ankle, knee and C-spine rules. There is also good guidance from the Royal

College of Radiology on the appropriate use of x-rays. However, the decision is ultimately a clinical judgement taking into account the mechanism of injury, examination factors and patient factors such as age.

Computed tomography (CT) scanning

Although seldom a first-line investigation, CT scanning is very good at providing detail in complex bony injury, for example complex mid-foot fractures and dislocations. It also may be necessary to image areas that are technically difficult such as the lower cervical spine.

Ultrasound and MR scanning

There are very few indications for immediate scanning in soft tissue problems. Exceptions would be suspected spinal cord compression. However, where an injury is not responding as it should to first-line management, and where clinical re-assessment indicates a significant problem, further imaging is indicated.

Other tests

In non-injury presentations there is a large variety of tests that might be indicated. For example, a patient presenting with shoulder-tip pain with no history of trauma may need one or more of the following: an electrocardiogram (ECG), chest x-ray, plain x-ray of the shoulder, a C-reactive protein (CRP or erythrocyte sedimentation rate (ESR), a pregnancy test, a CT abdomen and amylase. We are not advocating a barrage of tests on any one patient; this list is to illustrate the breadth of diagnosis that might be encountered. The selection of tests is wholly dependent on the clinical evaluation.

Patients on warfarin can present a problem. In the presence of excessive pain or swelling, check an International Ratio (INR).

Types of injury and treatment

Muscle body

Muscle body tears are common. The medial head of the gastrocnemius, hamstrings and biceps are particularly prone to this type of injury. They are usually caused by contraction against resistance. Most of these tears are not complete and settle with advice, initial rest and then graded rehabilitation including gentle stretching. Complete tears are more likely in the tendon or at bony origins and insertions. In very athletic individuals or those with high occupational demands careful follow up and perhaps further imaging might be indicated.

Direct blows or a muscle tear can cause a haematoma. These are mostly treated conservatively. It is important not to overstretch the muscle during healing or myositis ossificans might result.

One of the most serious muscle problems is compartment syndrome. Muscles are contained within myofascial envelopes that are relatively non-expandable. Any condition that results in swelling within the compartment (direct trauma, muscle tear, ischaemia) may result in an increase in the pressure within the compartment leading to ischaemia and eventual muscle death. *The* symptom of compartment syndrome is severe pain, often unresponsive to opiates and seemingly out of proportion to the severity of the injury. The sign of compartment syndrome is severe pain at rest and on passive muscle stretch.

Tendon/muscle origin and insertion

Tendon injuries tend to be more severe than muscle belly problems. Tears are often complete and more commonly require surgical intervention, especially in sportsmen or those with high occupational demands. These can be difficult to diagnose and if an injury is not settling then further imaging may be required. Sometimes a tear can pull off a piece of the bony attachment. An x-ray might be diagnostic but often ultrasound or MR are required. See Table 1.3.

Ligament

Ligament injuries are very common but represent a spectrum of injury from being minor and self-limiting to those that result in a mechanically unstable joint. The classification of these injuries into grade 1/2/3 tears is an inexact science but is a useful concept to emphasize the need to make some type of assessment of the severity of ligament injury (see Figure 1.8).

Taking the example of the lateral ligament of the ankle, a grade 1 tear would be a partial tear of one component of the lateral ligament complex, a stable injury that will resolve with conservative management. A grade 2 tear would be a complete tear of the anterior talo-fibular ligament, usually a stable injury but requiring more intensive follow up and management. A grade 3 tear would be a complete tear of the whole lateral ligament complex, an unstable injury that would require careful follow up, perhaps further imaging and consideration of a surgical repair. However, it is difficult to grade these injuries by clinical assessment alone, especially at the time of injury.

Functional impairment

One of the commonest problems with soft tissue injury is the loss of mobility, muscle bulk and slowing of protective reflexes caused

Table 1.3 Tendon tears that may require surgical treatment.

Tears at insertion	Tears in tendon	Tears at origin
Biceps insertion to radius at elbow	Extensor pollicis longus at wrist	Long head of biceps
Flexor digitorum profundus to the distal phalanx	Quadriceps tendon	Hamstrings at the ischial tuberosity
	Patellar tendon	Biceps femoris at the anterior inferior iliac spine
	Achilles tendon	
	Tibialis posterior tendon	

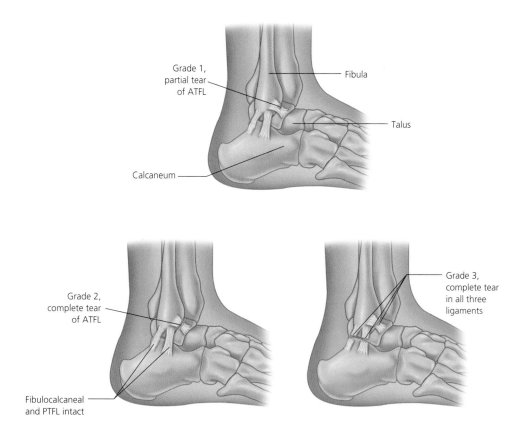

Figure 1.8 Grading of ligament tears. (a) Grade 1, a partial tear of part of the ligament complex (partial tear of the anterior talo-fibular ligament; ATFL). (b) Grade 2, complete tear of part of the ligament (complete tear of ATFL). (c) Grade 3, complete tear of the whole ligament complex (tears of the ATFL, calcaneo-fibular ligament and posterior talo-fibular ligament, PTFL).

by non-use or immobilization of an injured area. For example, the quadriceps muscle visibly losses bulk within a few days of the knee being immobilized. Given the importance of muscle power and reflexes in the maintenance of joint stability (see above), patients often report a feeling of insecurity, and 'giving way'. Equally strong muscles and fast reflexes can compensate for significant ligament tears, for example anterior cruciate injury.

Functional (rather than mechanical) instability is treated by rebuilding muscle bulk and retraining reflexes by intensive physiotherapy.

Joint injury

Dislocation

Dislocation is a serious injury as it always results in damage to the supporting ligaments. The shoulder and the fingers are the most common dislocations. Diagnosis is usually straightforward and treatment is by reduction, early support and then mobilization and rehabilitation.

Instability and recurrent dislocation

Instability is a common symptom. The commonest problem is functional instability due to muscle weakness (see above). Treatment is by good physiotherapy to build up muscle strength and protective reflexes. Recurrent dislocation indicates major damage to supporting structures and will require full investigation and in some cases surgery.

Loose body

Torn menisci, degenerative osteochondral fragments, osteochonditis and osteochondral fractures may all result in loose bodies within the joint. The commonest symptoms are pain, locking and giving way. Locking is where the patient says they are suddenly unable to move a joint through the full range of movement. Usually it is one specific movement that is blocked (e.g. in a truly locked knee the patient is unable to fully extend the knee but can flex well). Pseudo-locking, where a patient reports a global reduction in movement, is often due to pain inhibition or a joint effusion.

The other symptom is giving way, where the joint suddenly and completely fails. In the case of the knee the patient falls to the ground. True giving way is not common; functional giving way due to muscle weakness or pain inhibition usually does not result in total joint failure but more a 'feeling' of instability.

Nerve injury/compression

In closed injury it is uncommon for a nerve to be severed. The main mechanisms of injury are compression or stretching of the nerve fibres. Such injury can occur at the nerve roots (e.g. radiculopathy due to intervertebral disc disease), nerve plexus (e.g. traction brachial plexus injury) or in the peripheral nerve (e.g. radial nerve compression in the mid arm). A list of the common nerve injuries are given in Table 1.4.

Non-injury diagnosis and treatment

Limb pain with no definite single episode of injury is very common. The majority of these patients will have diagnoses that are not serious and most will resolve with good advice and simple treatments. However, sometimes a seemingly routine presentation will be the start of a serious condition where prompt diagnosis, referral and treatment may be life- or limb-saving (see Table 1.2 for the spectrum of injury in non-traumatic musculoskeletal problems).

Non-articular rheumatism

This is a spectrum of disease ranging from the common aches and pains that are experienced by almost all people at some time in their lives, such as mechanical back pain and cramp, through to serious conditions such as polymyalgia rheumatica (PMR). PMR is an inflammatory condition affecting the older population (peak incidence in the early 70s). The classical presentation is of shoulder and hip girdle pain and stiffness.

The major red flag for this condition is the association with giant cell arteritis. While not common, patients with symptoms of headache with PMR require urgent referral.

The management of mechanical back pain, fibromyalgia and muscle aches is covered in Chapter 3. However, the mainstays of treatment are encouraging mobility, exercise and simple analgesia.

Arthopathy
Degenerative arthopathy

Commonly known as osteoarthritis, this is the commonest joint problem. There is a spectrum of disease from mild single joint symptoms to severe multi-joint disease. Treatment aims at maintaining mobility and muscle strength along with measures to reduce load across the joint, such as weight reduction.

Autoimmune/reactive diseases

This is a large and diverse group of diseases including rheumatoid, psoriatic, enteropathic, juvenile arthritis and Reiter's disease. There tends to be multi-joint involvement. These patients need a detailed history and often extensive investigations to reach the definitive diagnosis leading to specific treatment. Referral to a rheumatologist is often required.

Crystal arthopathy

Gout (uric acid) and pseudogout (calcium pyrophosphate) arthopathy are common emergency presentations. The presentation of a hot red, painful joint often raises the possibility of sepsis. However, a careful history often reveals previous attacks or risk factors such as excess alcohol consumption or use of certain classes of drugs, obesity and metabolic syndrome. Pseudogout is much more common in the elderly. There are some typical presentations allowing a clinical diagnosis in well, apyrexial patients, for example acute pain and swelling in the first metatarso-phalangeal joint , wrist pain, swelling and erythema in an elderly patient with typical x-ray changes.

Acute attacks respond very quickly to anti-inflammatory drugs or steroids (colchicine is an alternative).

Septic arthopathy

Rightly feared as a diagnosis not to miss, septic arthritis is a limb- and occasionally life-threatening condition that requires fast and accurate diagnosis. The classical presentation is a hot, painful joint. Fever is not always present. The presentation may be atypical. If there is diagnostic doubt then the joint should be aspirated and sent for urgent microscopy and culture. Refer all patients with suspected septic arthritis to rheumatology or orthopaedics.

Diabetic arthopathy

Diabetic arthopathy is more common in older patients with type 1 diabetes and probably due to a number of factors such as micro-vascular disease, neuropathy and abnormal collagen formation. The hands, shoulders and feet are most commonly involved.

Neuropathic arthopathy

Normal proprioception and input from muscle, ligament and joint capsule coupled with good muscle reflexes are essential for normal joint function. Disruption of these functions lead to abnormal joint mechanics that eventually leads to severe joint destruction (Charcot joint). Commonest causes are diabetes, alcohol excess, spinal cord or central nervous system injury. These conditions require specialist referral.

Overuse syndromes

A sudden increase in activity or chronic repeated excess loading of the musculoskeletal system can lead to fractures (stress fracture),

Table 1.4 Nerve root and peripheral nerve injuries.

Nerve	Cause
Spinal nerve root	Compression from prolapsed disc or osteophytes
Brachial plexus injury	High velocity injury, abduction inury
T1 root	Thoracic outlet syndrome
Radial nerve	Compression in radial groove (Saturday night palsy)
Axillary nerve	Shoulder dislocation
Long thoracic nerve	Carrying heavy rucksack, blows to this area
Ulnar nerve, elbow	Compression behind lateral epicondyle
Ulnar nerve, wrist	Cycling
Anterior interosseus	Compression in upper forearm
Posterior interosseus	Compression in upper forearm
Median nerve	Carpal tunnel compression
Lateral cutaneous nerve thigh	Compression near the anterior superior iliac spine
Common peroneal nerve	Blow/fracture fibular head
Tibial nerve	Compression in tarsal tunnel

tendonitis, enthesiopathy, ligament failure and nerve compression. The level of activity in work/sport/hobbies is a vital part of the history and often is the major pointer to the diagnosis of these conditions. Treatment requires understanding of the biomechanics of the stresses involved, temporary reduction of aggravating factors and physiotherapy advice and education on how to avoid the problem in the future.

Tumour/pathological fractures

While these diagnoses are rare they should be kept in mind where the history is atypical (sudden onset of bone pain with no trauma) or common symptoms fail to improve or get worse (e.g. knee pain in a young individual). Where the patient has a known history of cancer you should have a low threshold for further investigation. The diagnosis with no such history can be difficult. The onset of symptoms is gradual and often indistinguishable from common conditions. There are a number of red flag symptoms that should increase the index of suspicion but these may be unreliable. Older patients, steroid use and history of cancer are the most useful pointers.

Complex regional pain syndrome/neural pain

In this condition there are abnormal vascular and neural reactions. There is often an episode of trauma, often minor. The symptoms are signs are grouped into sensory, vasomotor, sudomotor/oedema and motor/trophic categories. Treatments include patient education, drug treatment, rehabilitation and psychological support. Early referral to a specialist in this area is recommended.

Further reading

Brukner P, Khan K. *Clinical sports medicine*, 4th edn. McGraw-Hill Australia, North Ryde, NSW, 2012.

Davidovits P. *Physics in biology and medicine*, 3rd edn. Elsevier, Burlington MA, 2008.

McNeill AR. *The human machine*. Natural History Museum Publications, London, 1992.

Wardrope J, English B. *Musculo-skeletal problems in emergency medicine*. Oxford University Press, Oxford, 1998.

CHAPTER 2

Soft Tissue Problems of the Neck

Michael Athanassacopoulos and Neil Chiverton

Sheffield Teaching Hospitals NHS Foundation Trust, Sheffield, UK

OVERVIEW

- Whiplash-associated disorders (WADs) are very common and are cited in 85% of all claims of personal injury.

- WAD is an acute, self-limiting injury and the symptoms will subside within 4–6 weeks. Movement and activity within the patient's tolerance should be encouraged. There is no evidence to support the use of a collar.

- The most common presentation of acute torticollis is a patient aged 14–30 who wakes up with neck pain and deformity with significant muscle spasm, with a history of minor trauma or infection. An open-mouth odontoid view is the most useful initial investigation. Magnetic resonance imaging (MRI) is indicated in cases of a persistent painful torticollis to exclude less frequent causes.

- The majority of acute torticollis that occurs for less than 1 week is usually self-limiting and symptoms are managed with a combination of analgesia and physiotherapy.

- Cervical disc degeneration is a normal process of ageing. Symptoms may be acute or chronic; there may be axial pain, radicular compression or myelopathy.

- Progressive neurological deficit or acute deterioration necessitates an urgent referral. Persistence of arm pain after a trial of conservative treatment requires a non urgent referral. An emergency referral should be made in cases of sudden onset myelopathy, with an urgent referral in more chronic forms.

Whiplash-associated disorders

The term whiplash has been traditionally used to describe the neck injury that results from a sudden acceleration or deceleration that is not associated with fractures or dislocations of the cervical spine. Many other terms have been coined for this clinical syndrome, such as cervical strain or sprain, acceleration-deceleration syndrome and whiplash injury. In 1995 the Quebec Task Force (QTF; Spitzer *et al.* 1995) adopted the following definition: 'whiplash is an acceleration-deceleration mechanism of energy transfer to the neck. The impact may result in bony or soft tissue injuries, which in turn may lead to a variety of clinical manifestations named whiplash-associated disorders (WADs)'.

Incidence

The incidence is high estimated at 250 000 cases per year in the UK and 1 million in the USA. It is more common in those with pre-traumatic neck pain, low education level and female gender. Women are also more likely to suffer from chronic symptoms. In the UK 85% of all claims of personal injury are related to WAD. It is has been well documented to occur in low-velocity motor vehicle crashes (rear or side impact), and it can also occur following diving or actions that involve hyperextension and/or hyperflexion forces. In multiple trauma patients following high-energy accidents its incidence is 13%, similar to that of neck pain in the general population.

Etiology

The exact pathophysiology of WAD is not clear. Cadaveric studies have shown a complex movement differential of the upper and lower cervical spine, forming an S-shaped curve with muscles contracting in an attempt to stabilize the head. The change in velocity required to cause symptoms appears to be around 8 km/hour. The best available evidence points to the facet joint as the source of pain.

Clinical picture

The most common symptoms of pain and stiffness are related to the neck and the upper thoracic area. Most patients have no symptoms in the initial few minutes after the impact but these gradually intensify over the next few hours and days. There may be tinnitus, dizziness and blurred vision. The Quebec Task Force also developed a classification that is still in use with some modifications (Table 2.1). Grade 4 is sometimes excluded from WAD by some authors since it involves a fracture or dislocation. This classification is too simplified and does not adequately classify patients to aid in the clinical decision making. A subdivision of grade 2 has been proposed (Table 2.2).

Imaging

WAD diagnosis can be made clinically in most cases but imaging may be necessary to exclude more severe injuries. Several protocols

ABC of Common Soft Tissue Disorders, First Edition.
Edited by Francis Morris, Jim Wardrope and Paul Hattam.
© 2016 John Wiley & Sons, Ltd. Published 2016 by John Wiley & Sons, Ltd.

Table 2.1 Quebec Task Force classification of WAD.

WAD classification grade	Clinical presentation
Grade 0	No symptoms or signs
Grade 1	Neck symptoms (pain, stiffness and tenderness); no neck signs
Grade 2	Neck symptoms + neck signs (decreased range of motion and point tenderness)
Grade 3	Neck symptoms + neck signs + arm symptoms and signs (heaviness, fatigue, paraesthesia, weakness, decreased tendon reflexes)
Grade 4	Neck symptoms + neck signs + arm symptoms and signs + cervical fracture and/or dislocation

Table 2.2 Proposed subdivision of WAD grade 2.

WAD grade 2 subdivision	Clinical presentation
2A	Neck symptoms + neck signs (decreased range of motion, altered muscle recruitment patterns) + sensory impairment (local cervical mechanical hyperalgia)
2B	Neck symptoms + neck signs + sensory impairment + psychological impairment (elevated psychological distress)
2C	Neck symptoms + neck signs (decreased range of motion, altered muscle recruitment patterns, increased joint positioning errors) + sensory impairment (local cervical mechanical hyperalgia, generalized sensory hypersensitivity (mechanical, thermal, bilateral upper limb neurodynamic test 1 limitation); some may show sympathetic nervous system disturbances) + psychological impairment (elevated psychological distress, elevated levels of acute post-traumatic stress)

have been formulated for 'clearing the cervical spine' of more severe injuries without imaging. The most widely used is the Canadian Cervical Spine ('C-Spine') Rule algorithm for clearing the C-spine (Figure 2.1).

Treatment

Movement and activity within the patient's tolerance should be encouraged, but overstraining the painful structures of the neck should be avoided. Advise frequent short doses of exercise and activity throughout the day. There is consistent evidence that soft or rigid collars alone or in combination with other treatments are not associated with improvement of pain or disability in the short or long term. Analgesia is advised: non-steroidal anti-inflammatory drugs significantly reduce the disabling symptoms and total number of sick days. Psychological support may also be necessary.

Prognosis

In most cases WAD is a self-limiting injury. The symptoms will subside within 4–6 weeks, but 14–42% have persistent ongoing pain and 10% report constant pain. Factors associated with poor prognosis are pre-traumatic neck pain, low education level, older age, post-traumatic stress symptoms, female gender and WAD grades 2–3. Reduced range of motion and psychological disorder 3 months after the injury are predictors of persistent pain and disability. Symptoms persisting for more than 6 months are referred to by some authors as chronic whiplash.

Acute torticollis

Torticollis is Latin for twisted neck and is a symptom that can be caused by many pathological processes. The neck is laterally flexed and rotated towards the contralateral side. It can be classified as congenital (Figure 2.2), which is not painful, and acquired, which may or may not be painful (Table 2.3). It is outwith the scope of this chapter to discuss congenital and non-painful torticollis.

Clinical picture

By far the most common presentation is of idiopathic torticollis (wry neck; Figure 2.3). A typical case is a patient aged 14–30 who wakes up with neck pain and deformity with significant muscle spasm. The exact pathology is not clear but probably is due to a facet joint problem or sometimes a prolapsed disc.

Check that there is no history of trauma or infection, e.g. upper respiratory tract or retropharyngeal abscess, or ear nose and throat (ENT) procedures such as tonsillectomy. Ask if the patient has rheumatoid arthritis. These conditions can cause atlantoaxial rotatory subluxation (ARS). The onset of the torticollis in ARS this condition can be acute or appear even weeks after the insult. In post-traumatic cases the inciting incident may be very subtle and even unnoticed. It is believed that any inflammatory insult in this area may produce hyperemia in the ligaments of the atlantoaxial complex, which in turn leads to laxity and subluxation. If the subluxation and the original insult are left untreated a rigid deformity may develop.

Torticollis due to ARS is much more common in children. Characteristically the contralateral sternocleidomastoid muscle will be prominent due to the presence of spasm, as if trying to correct the deformity, which is the opposite to the congenital variant.

Imaging

In a typical case of wry neck that presents within 1–2 days after onset of symptoms an investigation is not usually required. However, if the symptoms are prolonged, the patient is a child or there are suspicions of trauma or recent infections, x-rays should be obtained. An open-mouth odontoid view is most useful in this case. In ARS there is rotation of C1 onto C2 and subluxation (Figure 2.4). If there is suspicion of these signs in the radiographs, then further imaging is indicated. A computed tomography (CT) scan should be obtained of the C1–C2 junction with the head rotated to the right and to the left by around 15°. This will show the absence of correction on turning of the head.

In atypical cases and those where symptoms are not settling a magnetic resonance (MR) scan may be indicated to exclude less frequent causes of torticollis such as infections or tumours.

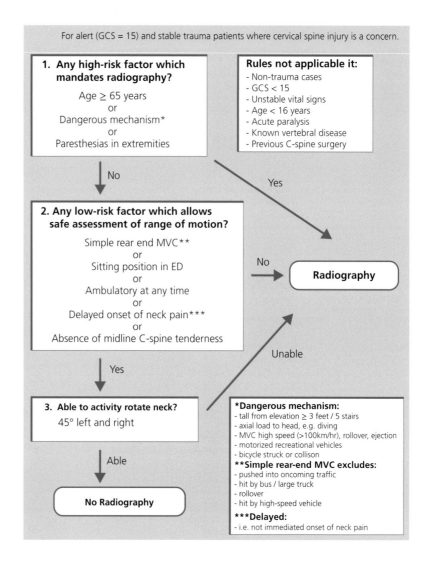

For alert (GCS = 15) and stable trauma patients where cervical spine injury is a concern.

1. Any high-risk factor which mandates radiography?

Age ≥ 65 years
or
Dangerous mechanism*
or
Paresthesias in extremities

Rules not applicable it:
- Non-trauma cases
- GCS < 15
- Unstable vital signs
- Age < 16 years
- Acute paralysis
- Known vertebral disease
- Previous C-spine surgery

No → Yes →

2. Any low-risk factor which allows safe assessment of range of motion?

Simple rear end MVC**
or
Sitting position in ED
or
Ambulatory at any time
or
Delayed onset of neck pain***
or
Absence of midline C-spine tenderness

No → **Radiography**

Unable →

Yes →

3. Able to activity rotate neck?
45° left and right

*Dangerous mechanism:
- tall from elevation ≥ 3 feet / 5 stairs
- axial load to head, e.g. diving
- MVC high speed (>100km/hr), rollover, ejection
- motorized recreational vehicles
- bicycle struck or collison
**Simple rear-end MVC excludes:
- pushed into oncoming traffic
- hit by bus / large truck
- rollover
- hit by high-speed vehicle
***Delayed:
- i.e. not immediated onset of neck pain

Able →

No Radiography

Figure 2.1 The Canadian Cervical Spine Rule algorithm for clearing the C-spine. ED, emergency department; GCS, Glasgow Coma Score; MVC, motor vehicle collision.

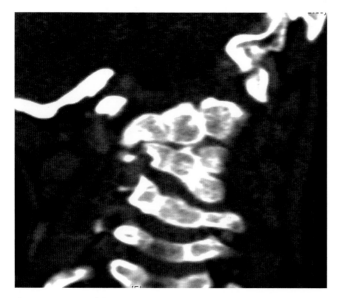

Figure 2.2 C1–C2 fully segmented hemivertebra on the left, causing congenital torticollis.

Treatment

In a typical case wry neck is treated with analgesia, muscle relaxants and physiotherapy. In the vast majority of cases the condition is self-limiting with symptoms settling after 7–10 days. Refer atypical cases, children, the elderly and those where a history might suggest a more serious condition.

In ARS, the treatment largely depends on the duration of symptoms and the persistence of deformity prior to seeking attention. The treatment varies from analgesics and observation to traction and manipulation to operative reduction and stabilization.

Cervical disc degeneration and related conditions

Cervical disc degeneration is a normal process of ageing. Trauma and repetitive motion may accelerate the condition. The prevalence of chronic neck pain (longer than 6 months in most studies) is approximately 10% in a large population. Cervical radiculopathy is less common and occurs in 0.5–3% of individuals, with a peak incidence around the age of 50.

Table 2.3 Differential diagnosis of painful torticollis.

Acute idiopathic (wry neck)

Traumatic	Atlantoaxial rotatory subluxation
	Os odontoideum
	C1 fracture
Inflammatory	Atlantoaxial rotator subluxation (Grisel's syndrome)
	Juvenile rheumatoid arthritis
	Discitis/osteomyelitis
	Other infection in neck
Tumours	Eosinophilic granuloma
	Osteoid osteoma/osteoblastoma
Cervical disc prolapse	
Sandifer's syndrome	

Acquired: painful or non-painful

Paroxysmal torticollis of infancy	
Tumour of the central nervous system	Posterior fossa
	Cervical cord
	Acoustic neuroma
Syringomyelia	
Hysterical	
Oculogyric crisis (phenothiazine toxicity)	
Associated with ligamentous laxity	Down syndrome
	Spondyloepiphyseal dysplasia/mucopolysaccharidosis

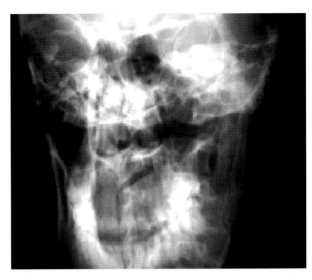

Figure 2.4 Anteroposterior radiogram focused on the upper C-spine of a patient with rotatory C1–C2 subluxation. Notice the difference in the distance between the two lateral masses of C1 and the odontoid process and the wink sign on the left. Due to the deformity and the pain it is frequently difficult to obtain proper open-mouth views.

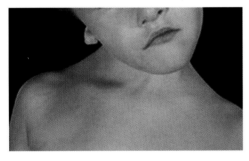

Figure 2.3 Photograph of a patient with torticollis due to C1–C2 hemivertebra. Notice the lateral flexion of the neck towards one side and the rotation towards the contralateral side.

Pathophysiology

The process of disc degeneration and sequelae have been summarized in Figure 2.5.

Clinical picture

The first symptoms of cervical disc degeneration are usually neck pain or stiffness. There may be associated irritation of the roots following leading to radiation of the pain. Irritation of the dorsal roots may radiate the pain on the occiput, shoulder or scapular areas (Figure 2.6a), while irritation of the ventral roots may radiate the pain on the ipsilateral arm on the corresponding dermatome (Figure 2.6b). A herniated disc pressing on the roots may also cause radicular pain with paraesthesia and less frequently weakness. If the central part of the canal is narrowed there may be symptoms of myelopathy with long tract signs affecting the legs.

History

There are a number of ways degenerative disease can present.

- There may be a sudden onset of neck and radicular pain which may be preceded by a trauma, accident, or lifting or pulling something, usually in younger patients. This is often due to a soft disc herniation.
- There may be a chronic history of symptoms due to spondylotic changes that is frequently multi-level, often with bilateral radiculopathy. This is often seen in older patients. In more central type of stenosis there may be a history of difficulty walking, clumsiness, writing or doing fine movements. This picture is usually chronic and slowly deteriorating.
- In 5% it can also be acute, usually following a trauma or a movement. This is usually seen in younger individuals with a large disc herniation or in patients with a marginally stenotic vertebral canal in which cases trauma can precipitate an acute myelopathic picture, leading to central cord syndrome.

The onset of symptoms and the exact distribution of pain and paraesthesia is noted. The patient should be asked specific questions, like: do you drop objects? Are you able to do up buttons? Has your handwriting changed? Such symptoms of muscle weakness may indicate myelopathy.

A general history should also be taken enquiring about previous cancer, any problems that might predispose to infection and the use of glucocorticoid medication that might indicate a cause other than degenerative changes.

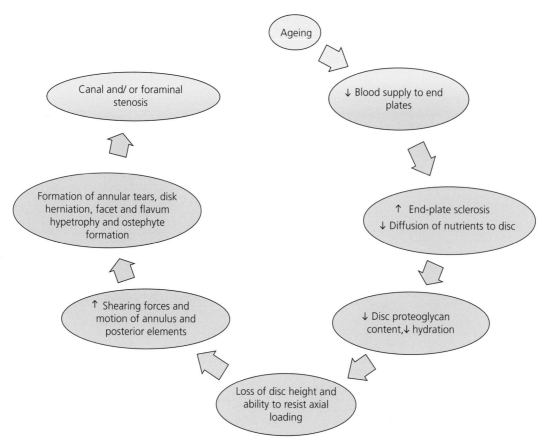

Figure 2.5 The pathophysiology of cervical disc degeneration.

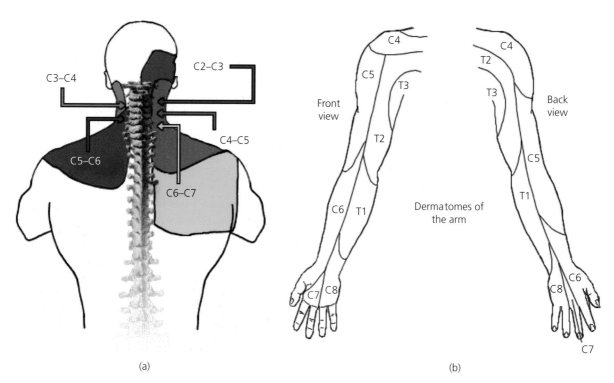

Figure 2.6 The dermatomes supplied by the (a) dorsal and (b) ventral cervical roots.

Examination

Observe the patient's gait. A characteristic wide, unsteady gait is seen in myelopathy. Feel the neck, noting areas and type of tenderness (e.g. severe tenderness to light touch). Finding a mass would be unusual but may denote the presence of a tumour or paraspinal abscess. Myofascial trigger points are commonly observed in the neck, parascapular region and upper back muscles of patients with cervical pathology. A recent study has shown that cervical root compression would be considered as the starting or maintaining factor of myofascial trigger points.

Ask the patient to move the neck gently through flexion, extension and lateral flexion, and rotation. Any triggered radicular or other symptoms should be noted.

A full sensory and motor assessment of the upper and *lower* limbs should be performed and documented. The presence of clonus, increased tone, hyper-reflexia and an upgoing plantar reflex are characteristic of myelopathy.

The Hoffmann sign is the upper extremity equivalent of the plantar reflex. It is elicited by stimulating the extensor tendon of the third digit with forceful flexion of the distal phalanx, followed by a sudden release. If there is a resultant flexion of the thumb, then the test is considered positive. A bilateral positive Hoffmann test can be normal but a unilateral positive test is always pathological.

The Lhermitte sign is the sensation of electric current along the spine during active flexion and extension. Spurling sign is when, during compression of the spine, lateral flexion and rotation leads to narrowing of the intervertebral foraminae, giving rise to ipsilateral radicular symptoms.

If the head is laterally flexed and rotated and the contralateral arm pulled, radicular symptoms may appear on the side of the pulled arm. This is because the root is fixed by the presence of a lateral hernia and cannot move while it is put under tension by pulling the arm and the head in opposite directions. Shoulder abduction reduces tension and shifts the nerve root away from sites of compression.

The inverted radial reflex is elicited by stimulating the brachioradialis tendon with gentle tapping. Hyperactive finger flexion is considered positive. The finger escape sign is evaluated by having the patient hold their fingers extended and adducted. If the ulnar digits drift into abduction within 30–60 seconds then the test is considered positive.

However, hyper-reflexia or provocative signs (Hoffmann, inverted radialis reflex, clonus, Babinski) are absent in up to 20% of patients with cervical myelopathy. Thus, the correlation of history, signs, symptoms and imaging will determine the diagnosis.

Imaging

X-rays should not routinely be performed in patients with neck pain. They should, however, be performed in cases of trauma or if a deformity, instability or congenital variations are suspected. They remain an important screening tool, are inexpensive and are easily obtained if symptoms are prolonged or if there are neurological signs. Flexion/extension films can uncover instability in segments that may be a cause of motion-induced pain. They are the only readily available dynamic way of imaging that can also show the effects of gravity since they can be taken on a standing position.

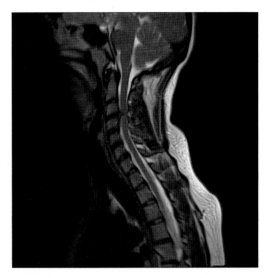

Figure 2.7 MR scan, sagittal section showing disc prolapse at C3/4 with compression of the spinal cord.

If the history and the examination are suggestive of significant cervical spine pathology then the ideal examination is a magnetic resonance imaging (MRI) scan (Figure 2.7). However, MRI changes can very frequently be seen in asymptomatic individuals. In a study of 30 asymptomatic individuals 73% showed bulging discs and 50% had focal disc protrusions. Also, degenerative disc disease may be found in 25% of asymptomatic patients under 40 and 60% of those older than 40. MRI results must be interpreted judiciously and closely correlated with symptoms and clinical examination.

Other imaging modalities like a CT scan or a CT myelogram are useful in cases of history of trauma or inability to have an MRI. They are less informative regarding the soft tissues. Neurophysiological studies are not usually needed in patients with a clinical picture of cervical radiculopathy and confirmatory imaging. However, they may be needed to differentiate cervical radiculopathy from peripheral nerve compression. Radiculopathy and peripheral nerve compression may co-exist (double crush phenomenon); for example, the presence of cervical disc herniation with carpal tunnel syndrome. The distal compression may greatly improve the clinical picture.

Treatment

The treatment of cervical pain without other symptoms is almost exclusively conservative. There is little medical evidence to support the use of cervical fusion or other surgical treatments for the treatment of axial neck pain.

Physiotherapy is the mainstay of management. Stretching should be performed early in the course of therapy. Daily stretching is optimal. This should be gentle and used as a warm up for a strength training routine. If manual therapy and exercise are combined there appears to be an additive effect.

Ultrasound, massage, transcutaneous nerve stimulation (TENS) and electrical stimulation have not been proven effective but some patients may find them useful. Acupuncture has been shown to have some short-term benefit, decreasing the need for analgesics. Injections of trigger points with local anaesthetics, steroids or dry needling have been done with equal effectiveness. Root injections, due to the severity of the complications, are rarely used and mostly for diagnostic purposes.

Psychological support in the form of advice, explanation, patient education and reassurance is the first line. Patients need to be clear that (a) although movement may hurt, this does not mean that damage is occurring, (b) they should return to work (or usual activities) even if the pain is not completely resolved, (c) they should use regular analgesics and (d) they may need to modify duties at work for a limited period. Self-management is emphasized throughout. A return to normal activities is encouraged.

Regular analgesics and a non-steroidal anti-inflammatory agent are preferred. Opioids constitute the second line. The use of muscle relaxants is appropriate if muscular spasm is present but use beyond 2 weeks is not advisable. Antidepressants may be of value as adjuvant analgesics for chronic neck and/or radicular pain, particularly in patients with associated sleep disorders and in those with catastrophizing psychology, anxiety or depression. Anticonvulsants, like gabapentin and pregabalin, have been used for radicular symptoms.

Soft cervical collars were shown to reduce pain in 76% of patients in a study in 1991 without affecting the range of motion. Their benefit may be just symptomatic, but there is no evidence of effect in the long-term outcome. Soft collars therefore are not generally advised but not contraindicated and can be used for a limited time, 2–3 weeks, but isometric neck exercises are recommended during use.

The treatment of cervical radiculopathy is multi-modal. It includes psychological, pharmacological and physiotherapy input, with surgical treatments reserved for the severe, the deteriorating and – possibly – the persistent cases. No single modality by itself is the answer. Multi-modal therapy that is customized to the patient is most likely to be successful.

At least 90% of patients with radiculopathy will recover without surgery. Surgical treatment is indicated in the presence of progressive neurological deficit, acute deterioration or persistence of arm pain after a trial of conservative treatment. Large disc herniations on imaging studies are not necessarily an indication for surgery. There is not a good correlation between imaging studies and symptoms. Even in patients with non-progressive weakness and minimal pain there is a good likelihood of resolution of the weakness without surgery.

The treatment of cervical myelopathy varies depending on the patient's age, severity of symptoms, level of ambulation and the diagnosis. Acute myelopathy from a disc herniation usually involves surgical decompression. In less acute cases, surgery should be reserved for those with progressive disability and those younger than age 60 years. Patients with mild disability are unlikely to worsen with conservative management but they may be at increased risk for spinal cord injury after minor trauma, which may support surgical treatment even in mild cases. Given the risks of surgery, these decisions should be taken by the patients in consultation with a spinal surgeon.

Prognosis

Risk factors for poorer outcomes in cervical radiculopathy include manual social class, catastrophizing, anxiety, depression, low treatment expectations, severity of baseline neck pain and disability, presence of comorbid back pain and age over 60 years. Another risk factor for poorer outcomes is a motor vehicle injury, with 20–70% of patients still symptomatic at 6 months. The patients with secondary gain were 9.5 times more likely to have long-term functional limitations.

In the majority of cases of cervical spondylotic myelopathy there is an initial phase of deterioration followed by a static period lasting a number of years, during which the degree of disability does not change significantly for those mildly affected. Moderate and severe cases tend to show progression.

Further reading

Baron E, Young W. Cervical spondylotic myelopathy: a brief review of its pathophysiology, clinical course, and diagnosis. *Neurosurgery* 2007;**60**(Suppl 1):S-35–S-41.

Foreman SM, Croft AC. *Whiplash injuries: the cervical acceleration/deceleration syndrome*, 3rd edn. Lippincott Williams & Wilkins, Baltimore, 2002.

Mazanec D, Reddy A. Medical management of cervical spondylosis. *Neurosurgery* 2007;**60**(Suppl 1):S43–S50.

Spitzer WO, Skovron ML, Salmi LR *et al.* Scientific monograph of the Quebec Task Force on Whiplash Associated Disorders: redefining "whiplash" and its management. *Spine* 1995;**20-8S**:1S–73S.

Sterling M. A proposed new classification system for whiplash associated disorders—implications for assessment and management. *Manual Ther* 2004;**9**:60–70.

Sterling M, Jull G, Kenardy J. Physical and psychological factors maintain long-term predictive capacity post-whiplash injury. *Pain* 2006;**122**:102–108.

Stiell IG, Wells GA, Vandemheen KL *et al.* The Canadian Cervical Spine Radiography Rule for alert and stable trauma patients. *J Am Med Assoc* 2001;**286**:1841–1848.

CHAPTER 3

Back Pain

Ben Cooper[1], Richard J. Follett[2] and Neil Chiverton[1]

[1]Sheffield Teaching Hospitals NHS Foundation Trust, Sheffield, UK
[2]Fit4-Physio, Sheffield, UK

OVERVIEW
- This chapter reviews the anatomy of the back.
- It reviews mechanical and non-mechanical causes of back pain.
- Also covered are cauda equina and red flags, and the systemic and psychological factors in back pain.

Introduction

Back pain is a major public health problem worldwide with the lifetime incidence of lower back pain reported to be as high as 84%. With back pain being such a significant clinical complaint it is important to understand how to assess and manage this condition and recognize those patients whose back pain is the result of serious pathology.

Types of back pain

Many attempts have been made to classify lower back pain but in general terms it can be divided into the following areas:

- mechanical; for example, degenerative disc disease,
- non-mechanical; for example, tumours,
- referred pain; for example, renal calculi,
- systemic or psychological; for example, fibromyalgia.

By far the most common cause of lower back pain is wear-and-tear change, which gives rise to 'mechanical' back pain. It is important to recognize how to elicit the signs and symptoms that would point you towards non-mechanical causes of pain.

Anatomy

The back is made up of 12 thoracic (T) and 5 lumbar (L) vertebrae which are separated by intervertebral discs. These discs act as the shock absorbers and are also important in facilitating normal back movements. The whole spine is stabilized by a number of ligaments, most importantly the anterior longitudinal ligament, which attaches to the anterolateral aspects of the vertebral bodies. The interspinous, supraspinous and posterior longitudinal ligaments along with the ligamentum flavum also contribute to stability, particularly in flexion. The facet joints and capsules also contribute to spinal stability. The muscular anatomy of a section of the spine is shown in Figure 3.1.

The most important anatomical relationship to remember is that of the spinal cord. The spinal cord ends at the level of T12/L1 and then becomes a mass of nerves that branch off from the lower end of the spinal cord, referred to as the cauda equina. It contains the nerve roots from L1–L5 and sacral (S)1–S4. The nerve roots from L4 to S4 join at the sacral plexus to form the sciatic nerve. Compression, trauma or other damage to this region of the spinal cord can result in cauda equina syndrome.

Thoracic back pain

Thoracic pain is commonly encountered and can provide a diagnostic challenge. Whereas mechanical disorders are most common, pain can emanate from visceral referral or non-mechanical causes. A careful history and examination must be taken to eliminate non-mechanical sources of pain before embarking on treatment.

Mechanical pain often originates from displacement of the costovertebral joints, which results in sudden-onset, unilateral pain combined with asymmetrical loss of trunk rotation movement. These problems are thought to arise because of the shallow articulations between the head of the rib and the vertebral body which renders them vulnerable to subluxation. Treatment by manipulation is very effective and the pain usually resolves within days. The relative rigidity of the thoracic spine due to sternal and vertebral articulations of ribs makes discal injury comparatively rare.

The clinician should be aware of other causes of pain such as discitis, malignancy (primary and secondary: bronchus, breast, kidney, prostate and thyroid), osteoporotic fractures, Scheurmann's disease, inflammatory arthritis and the viscera (heart, lung, pancreas and gall bladder all have the capacity to refer into the thorax). The cervical spine can also refer pain into the mid-thoracic area.

ABC of Common Soft Tissue Disorders, First Edition.
Edited by Francis Morris, Jim Wardrope and Paul Hattam.
© 2016 John Wiley & Sons, Ltd. Published 2016 by John Wiley & Sons, Ltd.

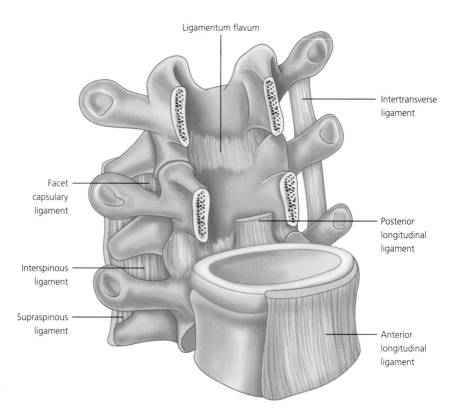

Ligamentum flavum

Intertransverse ligament

Facet capsulary ligament

Posterior longitudinal ligament

Interspinous ligament

Supraspinous ligament

Anterior longitudinal ligament

Figure 3.1 The muscular anatomy of a section of the spine.

Mechanical lower back pain

Commonly, a patient's first episode of mechanical back pain will be between the ages of 20 and 40 years. Whereas some describe pain after specific movements others describe the spontaneous onset of symptoms. The back pain is experienced in the lumbar region and referral to the buttocks, thighs and groin are common. Symptoms are typically provoked by flexion, lifting, twisting and sitting and are frequently worse in the morning. Movement and exercise may help relieve symptoms and the patient will have no red flags or neurology, as detailed below.

Cauda equina syndrome

This rare but important condition occurs most frequently as a consequence of a large lower lumbar disc sequestration, prolapse or herniation. It is usually characterized by the following:

- severe lower back,
- sciatica: sometimes bilateral or absent,
- saddle and/or genital sensory disturbance,
- bladder, bowel and sexual dysfunction.

This is surgical emergency and immediate referral to the on-call orthopaedic team is imperative for early examination, as is consideration for urgent magnetic resonance imaging (MRI) with or without surgical decompression.

Prolapsed intervertebral disc

The usual pattern of prolapse involves the tearing of the annulus of the disc that allows the semi-liquid nucleus pulposus to bulge.

This happens most commonly at the L5/S1 disc and frequently presses on a lumbar nerve route, causing pain and paraesthesiae to the leg in a segmental pattern and dependent on the level of the prolapse. MRI of prolapsed intervertebral disc is shown in Figure 3.2.

Non-mechanical and referred causes of back pain

Less commonly, back pain is the result of non-mechanical conditions such as those highlighted in Box 3.1. It is important to try to distinguish these pathologies from simple mechanical back pain with a thorough history and examination. Tumours that commonly metastasize to the spine are listed in in Box 3.2.

Box 3.1 **Serious pathologies associated with back pain**

- Malignancy (primary and secondary)
- Infection; for example, transverse myelitis/epidural abscess
- Spinal fracture from trauma
- Referred pain; for example, abdominal aortic aneurysm, renal calculi

Other causes of back pain to consider

- Spondylolisthesis
- Spinal stenosis
- Arthropathies; for example, ankylosing spondylitis
- Metabolic bone disease; for example, osteoporosis, Paget's disease

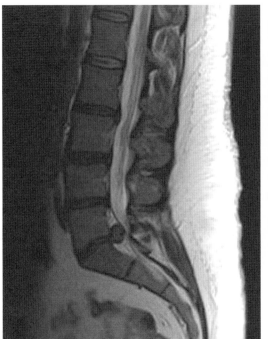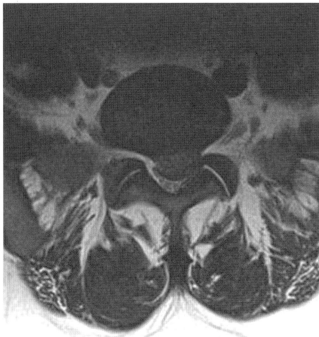

Figure 3.2 MRI of prolapsed intervertebral disc.

Red flags in back pain

Certain key indicators of serious spinal pathology need to be elicited during your history taking and examination. These indicators are sometimes referred to as the red flags of back pain. Specific red flags are listed in Box 3.3 and when present may indicate a more sinister cause for a patient's back pain rather than a purely mechanical pathology. Following assessment, if a serious spinal pathology is suspected then further investigation is warranted and should be tailored towards this suspected pathology.

Systemic and psychological factors in back pain

Successfully distinguishing specific and/or serious causes of back pain can be achieved with a good history and examination but trying to elicit whether non-specific mechanical back pain is genuine or a functional pain with significant psychological overlay can be trickier. Almost every patient presenting with back pain is likely to have already developed some attitudes and beliefs around their condition that ultimately may affect the outcome of their episode of impairment. The bio-psycho-social model for assessment of back pain highlights attitudes, behaviours and beliefs that are considered risk factors for chronicity and potential for long-term disability in those presenting with mechanical back pain. These are known as yellow flags of back pain and are summarized in Box 3.4. Physical examination techniques described in the literature attempt to highlight these factors but all have a very poor prognostic value. As a result, when in doubt the patient should be treated as having 'organic' back pain.

Fibromyalgia

Fibromyalgia is a fairly common long-term (chronic) condition that causes widespread muscular pain, including back pain. It affects women more than men and the condition varies a great deal from one person to another and from day to day. It is thought that the condition is a combination of physical, mental and psychological factors. Importantly, the condition is not inflammatory or degenerative so it will not have any lasting physical effects on a patient. However, it can have a major impact on quality of life and patients with back pain related to this condition may need a combination of analgesics, antidepressants, physiotherapy and occupational therapy.

History and examination

History

A full and thorough history and examination are important when assessing new episodes or exacerbations of back pain. Important points that need to be covered when taking a history are listed in Box 3.5. These questions help you make a diagnosis so that you may offer the patient appropriate treatment as well as helping to exclude the more sinister causes of back pain.

Examination

Every examination should include inspection of the spine, tests for range of movement and passive range-of-motion testing of the hips.

Finally, special testing and palpation are used to confirm findings appreciated earlier in the examination.

Look

Stand the patient up and inspect from the front, sides and rear, looking for any abnormal spinal or pelvic curvature, asymmetries in skin folds or muscle atrophy. When identified, symmetry of the spine and pelvis should be reassessed with the patient seated to correct for the discrepancies in leg length that may be the cause of pelvis or spinal asymmetry when standing.

Feel

Palpation of the lumbar spine should confirm the findings of the initial examination of movement and try to further locate where the pain is originating. Palpate the following with the patient seated or prone:

- spinous processes to check for bony tenderness and for deformity,
- muscles of the erector spinae and the transverse processes.

With the patient prone, examine:

- sacrum,
- sacroiliac joints,
- posterior superior iliac spine,
- piriformis.

And then, with the patient supine, examine:

- anterior superior iliac spine,
- anterior inferior iliac spine,
- pubic bone,
- abdomen.

Move

Examine the movement of the lumbar spine as follows:

- forward flexion,
- extension,
- lateral flexion (left and right),
- rotation (left and right),
- passive hip range of motion with the patient supine (note any asymmetry to attempt to exclude pathology of the hip joint, which may be confused with degenerative lumbar spinal conditions),
- normal gait.

Neurological

A full neurological examination of the lower limbs should be considered in all cases of lower back pain, in particular where pain radiates below the knee or where neurological symptoms are described by the patient. This should include examination of:

- myotomes (Table 3.1),
- dermatomes (Figure 3.3),
- reflexes with Babinski sign for signs of an upper motor lesion,
- coordination (Romberg's test, heel-to-toe walking),

Table 3.1 Myotomes.

Myotome	Action
L1, L2	Hip flexion
L3	Knee extension
L4	Ankle dorsiflexion
L5	Big toe extension
S1	Ankle plantarflexion
S2	Knee flexion

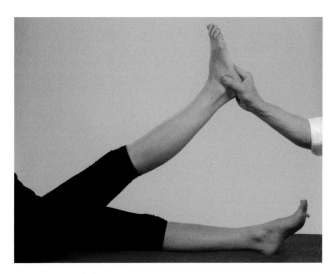

Figure 3.4 Straight leg raise.

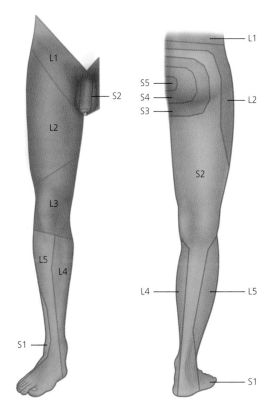

Figure 3.3 Dermatomes.

- rectal examination to assess tone and anal wink, in the context of any reported bladder or bowel dysfunction or saddle anaesthesia,
- perianal sensation,
- straight leg raise (Figure 3.4).

A straight leg raise is an important extra test to perform when examining a patient with back pain. This should consist of laying the patient supine and passively raising one leg with a straight knee until pain is elicited in any part of the leg or buttock. If their pain is provoked then lower the leg slightly and then dorsiflex the foot. This test is positive if it causes additional pain and can be relieved by flexing the knee.

Other examinations

Consider referred pain from abdominal pathology in patients with back pain, for example abdominal aortic aneurysm in the middle aged and elderly, and renal stone disease. Abnormal vital signs (fever, hypotension) in the presence of back pain are concerning and the cause is unlikely to be mechanical in nature.

Other examination techniques may be useful in identifying the source of back pain:

- muscle testing to evaluate the muscles supporting the spinal column for strength, stability and pain,
- stork stand test to evaluate for spondylolysis and/or sacroiliac dysfunction,
- the FABER test (flexion, abduction, external rotation of the hip) to evaluate for pathology of the sacroiliac joint and hip,
- the Trendelenburg test to evaluate for weak or injured gluteus medius and minimus muscles,
- reverse Lasegue test to look for high lumbar disc lesions.

Investigations

Common imaging investigations considered by clinicians are plain x-rays of the lumbar spine and MRI scans. There is also no evidence of a clinical benefit from referral for MRI compared to x-ray in terms of pain and disability. The only applicable benefit of MRI is to exclude cauda equina syndrome and in cases of non-specific lower back pain for identifying those patients who may benefit from surgery. In these patients, early MRI may improve outcomes and be cost-effective. Other specific investigations such as inflammatory markers or a bone scan should be considered in patients with red flags.

Treatment

When considering treatment options for back pain the treating clinician should take into account the patient's needs and wishes. In the short term, analgesia is usually required to provide initial relief of symptoms. Options to consider regarding analgesia are given in Box 3.6.

Educational advice regarding self-management of lower back pain and encouragement to stay active as much as possible is recommended as the treatment of choice for most patients with mechanical back pain. Referral to physiotherapy is useful in some cases. Physiotherapy treatment options include an exercise programme tailored to the person, which could include aerobic activity, movement instruction, muscle strengthening, postural control and stretching. Courses of manual therapy or acupuncture have also been shown to be of benefit for patients suffering from back pain. In a minority of cases a combination of physiological and physical treatments may be needed.

The prognosis for complete recovery in mechanical back pain is excellent. Within 6 weeks 90% of patients with both new and recurrent episodes of mechanical back pain are symptom-free. A further 5% recover within 12 weeks. The remaining 5% develop persistent pain leading to chronic lower back pain but this does not equate with disability and only in a small percentage of cases do psychological and psychosocial factors lead to a significant impact on a person's activities of daily living.

Only patients who still have severe non-specific lower back pain despite undergoing a full programme as outlined above should be referred for orthopaedic consultation should they wish to consider surgery. Remember that only 10% of patients with a herniated cervical disc require surgical treatment, and most people make a full recovery with conservative treatment alone.

Other treatment options, including laser therapy, interferential therapy, therapeutic ultrasound, transcutaneous nerve stimulation (TENS) and lumbar supports, have no good evidence to suggest that they are effective treatment options and should not be recommended. Likewise, intradiscal electrothermal therapy (IDET), percutaneous intradiscal radiofrequency thermocoagulation (PIRFT) and radiofrequency facet joint denervation should not be recommended.

Further reading

Balague F, Mannion AF, Pellisé F, Cedraschi C. Non-specific low back pain. *Lancet* 2012;**379**:482–491.

Department for Work and Pensions. Medical guidance for DLA and AA decision makers (adult cases): staff guide. http://www.dwp.gov.uk/publications/specialist-guides/medical-conditions/a-z-of-medical-conditions/back-pain/mech-back-pain.shtml (accessed 8 December 2015).

Gardner A, Gardner E, Morley T. Cauda equina syndrome; a review of the current clinical and medico-legal position. *Eur Spine J* 2011;**20**:690–697.

McRae R. *Pocket book of orthopaedics and fractures*, 2nd edn. Churchill Livingstone, Edinburgh, 2006.

Sandella BJ. Examination of low back pain. http://emedicine.medscape.com/article/2092651-overview (accessed 8 December 2015).

Samanta J, Kendal Jl, Samanta A. 10 minute consultation: chronic back pain. *BMJ* 2003;**326**:535.

Wardrope J, English B. *Musculo-skeletal problems in emergency medicine.* Oxford University Press, Oxford, 1998, pp. 296–297.

National Collaborating Centre for Primary Care. *Low back pain: early management of persistent non-specific low back pain.* Royal College of General Practitioners, London, 2009.

Sheffield Back Pain. Yellow flags in back pain. http://www.sheffieldbackpain.com/professional-resources/learning/in-detail/yellow-flags-in-back-pain (accessed 8 December 2015).

Arthritis Research UK. Fibromyalgia. http://www.arthritisresearchuk.org/arthritis-information/conditions/fibromyalgia.aspx (accessed 8 December 2015).

CHAPTER 4

Shoulder: Sub-acromial Pathology

Lennard Funk

Wrightington, Wigan & Leigh NHS Trust, Wrightington, UK

OVERVIEW

- The shoulder is not a joint, but a complex of muscles, ligaments and articulations that function to position the hand in space.
- The rotator cuff is a confluence of the deep muscles of the shoulder that stabilize and centre the humeral head for movement.
- Sub-acromial impingement may have direct space-occupying causes or may be secondary.
- The cause of the impingement should be sought and treated.
- Most degenerative rotator cuff tears can be managed non-operatively, but traumatic tears generally require surgical repair.
- Ultrasound scans are useful to detect tears, but magnetic resonance imaging can provide additional information on the quality of the muscles and associated pathologies.
- Acute calcific episodes can be extremely painful, requiring urgent treatment in the form of injections or surgery.
- Ultrasound scanning is the best investigation for detecting extra-articular proximal biceps pathologies.
- Biceps tendonitis can be treated with a tenotomy or tenodesis, depending on the age and functional demands of the patient.
- Most long head of biceps ruptures have an asymptomatic popeye deformity.

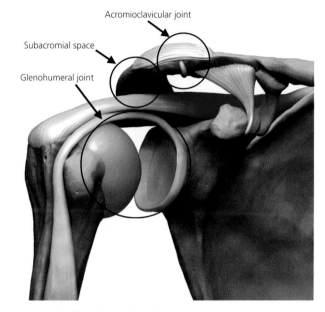

Figure 4.1 Shoulder joints and articulations.

acromion; covered in this chapter) and *articular* structures (including the articular labrum, the biceps, capsule and acromioclavicular joint; covered in Chapter 5). See Figure 4.1.

The rotator cuff

There are two layers of muscles that move the shoulder (see Figure 4.2). The *superficial* layer is made up of the large muscles (deltoid, pectoralis major, latissimus dorsi, teres major) that provide power and motion of the glenohumeral joint. The *deep layer* is a smaller group of muscles known as the rotator cuff (supraspinatus, infraspinatus, teres minor, subscapularis) that arise from the scapula and attach to the proximal humerus, merging and enveloping the humeral head. As a combined unit, they function to stabilize and secure the humeral head against the glenoid (i.e. 'cuff'), which in turn enables the large muscles to rotate (i.e. 'rotator') the humeral head and generate the forces needed for upper limb function.

Any injury or disease that causes dysfunction of the rotator cuff mechanism will unbalance this finely controlled system, leading to

The shoulder is the most mobile joint of the body providing strength and movement to the arm. It is not really a joint, but a complex of over 30 muscles, five joints and numerous ligaments. This 'shoulder complex' presents a compromise between stability and mobility, and the result is that it is inherently unstable. More than any other joint, its mobility and stability is controlled by muscles and tendons that in turn become prone to injury and disease. This can create diagnostic challenges but a good knowledge of the anatomy and biomechanics of the shoulder combined with a careful examination will help to isolate the likely cause of pain and dysfunction. The primary sources of pain originate from the *sub-acromial* area (incorporating the rotator cuff, the bursa and the

ABC of Common Soft Tissue Disorders, First Edition.
Edited by Francis Morris, Jim Wardrope and Paul Hattam.
© 2016 John Wiley & Sons, Ltd. Published 2016 by John Wiley & Sons, Ltd.

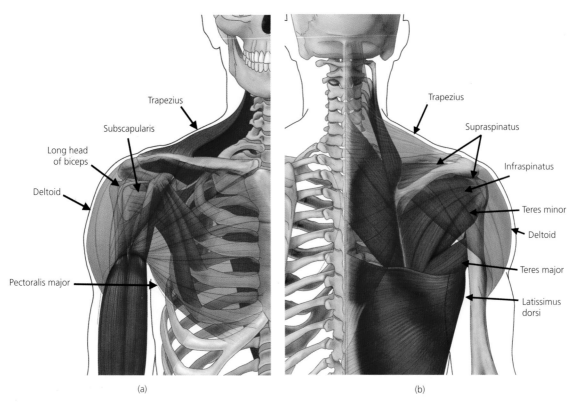

Figure 4.2 The superficial and deep muscle layers of the shoulder. (a) Anterior. (b) Posterior.

loss of control of the humeral head against the glenoid and abnormal movement patterns that can cause pain.

Sub-acromial impingement

The rotator cuff muscles work together to depress and centralize the humeral head in the glenohumeral joint. As the arm is elevated, the rotator cuff depresses the humeral head allowing it to rotate and glide easily underneath the acromion. Any injury or disorder of the rotator cuff impairs this mechanism. This in turn leads to abutment of the cuff against the undersurface of the acromion, causing 'impingement' of the rotator cuff and inflammation of the sub-acromial bursa, a fluid sac that reduces the friction of sub-acromial movements. See Box 4.1.

History and examination

Primary sub-acromial impingement usually affects people in their thirties to sixties. They have pain when raising their arm to shoulder height and overhead. Activities that involve this movement, particularly with internal rotation, are painful. This can include dressing, driving, grooming and pouring a kettle. Sleep can also be painful when lying on the affected shoulder.

Range of motion below shoulder height is not limited or painful, but abduction and elevation is limited by mid-arc pain. This is generally worse with the shoulder in internal rotation (thumb down). The positive clinical tests can include the following.

- Neer's sign: pain on passive abduction to mid range, with the arm fully internally rotated (Figure 4.4a).

Box 4.1 Causes of sub-acromial impingement

Primary: caused by pathology or injury to the cuff (usually in older age groups)

See Figure 4.3a.

- Rotator cuff strain
- Partial- or full-thickness tear
- Calcific tendonitis
- A tendonopathy due to chronic overuse

Secondary: caused by stability problems (usually in younger age groups)

See Figure 4.3b.

- Glenohumeral instability
- Labral tears (in particular superior labrum anteroposterior (SLAP) tears)
- Abnormal muscle patterning problems of the shoulder.

Structural: caused by narrowing of the sub-acromial space

- Acromial shape: differences in the shape of the acromium were described by Nicholson *et al.* (1996). Type I is flat, type II is curved and type III is hooked. A person with a type II or type III acromion would be at a higher risk of impingement due to the narrowing of the acromiohumeral gap and bursal space.
- Acromial spur: with advancing age people tend to develop a bone spur on the front and side of the acromion. This further reduces the sub-acromial space, increasing the risk of impingement.
- Acromio-clavicular joint (ACJ) arthritis: inferior osteophytes can 'impinge' on the underlying rotator cuff.

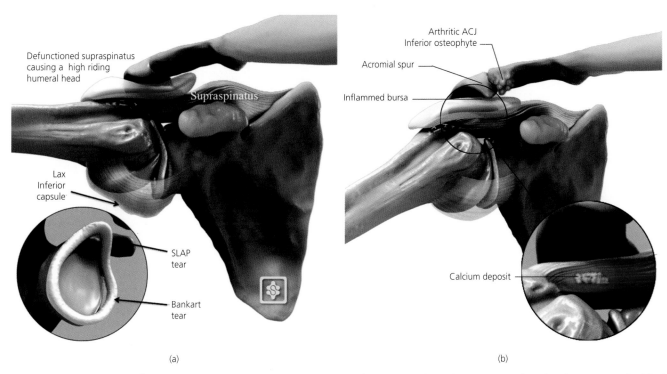

(a)

(b)

Figure 4.3 (a) Primary causes of impingement (older people). (b) Secondary causes of impingement (young). ACJ, acromio-clavicular joint; SLAP, superior labral anteroposterior.

- Copeland's impingement test: positive Neer's sign and then pain-free abduction with the arm fully externally rotated (Figure 4.4b).
- Hawkin's test: pain on passive internal rotation with the arm in flexion to 90° (Figure 4.4c).

Investigations

The diagnosis of sub-acromial impingement is based on the clinical history and examination findings. Investigations are not required to diagnose the impingement, but are necessary to find the cause of the impingement. The main investigations are:

- Plain radiographs: this should include anteroposterior, axillary and supraspinatus outlet views. Look for calcific tendonitis, acromioclavicular joint arthritis, large acromial spurs, acromial shape and the humeral head position in relation to the glenoid.
- Ultrasound scan: allows dynamic evaluation of the rotator cuff. Look for rotator cuff tears, calcific tendonitis, sub-acromial bursal fluid and the long head of biceps.
- MRI scan: not usually required, but can demonstrate rotator cuff pathology better than ultrasound scans. Worse than ultrasound and radiographs for calcific tendonitis.

Treatment

Treatment of impingement depends on the cause.

Physiotherapy

If the problem originates from injury to the rotator cuff (younger), a degenerative tendinopathy (older) or instability caused by a muscle patterning problem, most patients improve with physiotherapy and anti-inflammatory drugs. The aims of the physiotherapy treatment are to increase the sub-acromial space by improving shoulder posture and movement control and to progressively load the contractile structures with strengthening exercises, re-education and functional rehabilitation until normal function has been restored.

Non-steroidal anti-inflammatory drugs (NSAIDs) and injection therapy

Anti-inflammatories are required to reduce the swelling and pain of the sub-acromial bursa. If the pain is not severe this can be achieved with NSAIDs. However, if the pain is severe a corticosteroid injection into the sub-acromial bursa may be required. The injection provides sufficient pain relief to enable greater compliance and improved outcomes from physiotherapy. There is also some evidence that injections of hyaluronic acid preparations can reduce pain and facilitate recovery. Injections are of short-term benefit only and appropriate rehabilitation is essential following an injection. Over 70% of patients with primary sub-acromial impingement will recover with this approach.

Surgery

In resistant cases where injections and rehabilitation have failed, surgery may be required. Again, surgery will depend on the cause. If there is a narrow acromial space due to ACJ arthritis or calcific tendonitis or rotator cuff tears then these need to be addressed directly. If these have been excluded, then a sub-acromial decompression procedure is indicated. The surgery is usually performed arthroscopically and involves division of the coraco-acromial

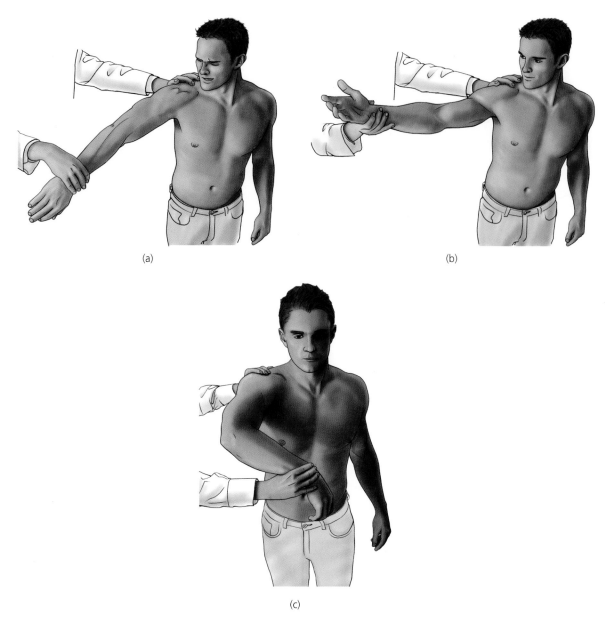

Figure 4.4 (a) Neer's sign. (b) Copeland's impingement test. (c) Hawkin's test.

ligament and flattening of the undersurface of the acromion. In these cases the success rate is over 80%.

Rotator cuff tears

Causes

In young adults and children the rotator cuff tendons are extremely tough and robust, but with age they degenerate and lose their strength. Genetic predisposition can affect the rate of cuff degeneration too. Degenerative tendon tearing is not uncommon with advancing age and is often asymptomatic. Rotator cuff tendons are prone to injury, which can lead from 'wear' to 'tear', where injury causes traumatic tissue failure and symptoms develop. The more degenerate a tendon is, the less trauma required to tear it.

History and examination

The classical history is a fall or wrenching injury to the shoulder with immediate pain. Progressive weakness is noticed and it is both painful and difficult to lift the arm. People often report having to use their opposite hand to assist the affected one with activities such as using a kettle. The clinical examination should reveal similar positive tests to impingement, although abduction and elevation may be limited by weakness, as well as pain.

Relevant tests for rotator cuff weakness involve isolating the component muscles of the rotator cuff to test them (see Figure 4.5).

Investigations

As for sub-acromial impingement, ultrasound is better for a dynamic assessment of the rotator cuff, but magnetic resonance

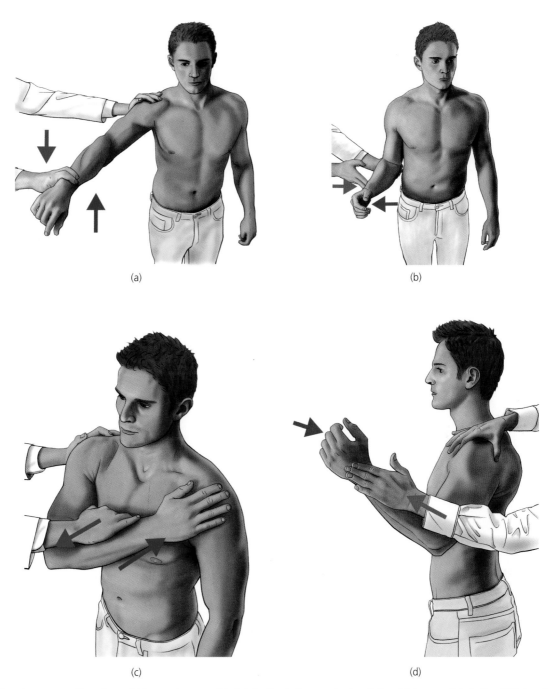

Figure 4.5 Tests for rotator cuff weakness. (a) Supraspinatus: resisted abduction in the scapula plane below 40 degrees of abduction. (b) Infraspinatus: resisted external rotation. (c) Subscapularis: resisted internal rotation. The 'bear hug' test. (d) Teres minor: resisted external rotation in abduction. Green arrows, examiner's force; red arrows, patient's resistance.

imaging (MRI) demonstrates the rotator cuff tear size, location and the quality and atrophy of the rotator cuff muscles.

Treatment

Traumatic rotator cuff tears in active people are best treated with surgical repair as soon as possible, since the tears increase in size and the muscle degenerates further with increasing time after injury. This is usually performed arthroscopically, with good success rates. *Atraumatic*, degenerative tears (wear) do not usually require a repair and can be treated in a similar way to sub-acromial impingement. If there is functional weakness, the 'deltoid rehabilitation' programme is undertaken to strengthen the deltoid muscle so it is able to compensate for the weakened rotator cuff and improve functional motion and strength.

If non-operative means fail to improve the pain, then surgery is required. This generally includes a sub-acromial decompression and possibly biceps tenotomy if the biceps is involved (which it often is). In a younger and active patient with higher functional demands a rotator cuff repair is associated with better strength gains compared to decompression alone, although the recovery time is longer and there is little difference in pain relief between the two.

Calcific tendonitis

Causes

The aetiology of calcific tendonitis is unknown. It tends to affect people in their mid-life between the ages of 30 to 60 years. The process follows three phases.

- Calcific phase: the deposition of calcium is not usually painful.
- The resting period: predominantly impingement pain.
- Resorptive phase: can be very painful, with release of calcium crystals into the sub-acromial bursa and/or glenohumeral joint.

The natural progression is for spontaneous resolution, with 85% of 'fluffy' deposits and 33% of dense deposits disappearing in 3 years.

History and examination

In the resting phase the clinical history and findings are identical to sub-acromial impingement. The severe pain of the resorptive phase is known as an *acute calcific event*. The pain is due to leakage of calcium crystals into the sub-acromial bursa or glenohumeral joint, where they cause an intense chemical inflammatory response.

Investigations

The calcific deposits can be seen on plain radiographs, as well as ultrasound scan. They often cannot be seen on standard MRI scans.

Treatment

Management is similar to sub-acromial impingement for patients in the resting phase, with physiotherapy and sub-acromial injections being the initial treatment. The severe pain of the acute calcific event warrants urgent treatment with sub-acromial corticosteroid injection, collar and cuff or sling support or even arthroscopic washout and release of the calcific deposit. The very acute symptoms do usually settle within 2–4 weeks but active management is essential as the pain will seriously impair sleep and basic daily function.

If conservative management fails, treatment options to encourage dissolution of the calcific deposit include the following.

- Ultrasound-guided barbotage: under ultrasound guidance the calcific deposit is either broken up and/or suctioned with a needle under local anaesthetic. Barbotage is quick, safe and minimally invasive with a success rate of over 70%.
- Extracorporeal shock wave therapy: the aim is to focus acoustic energy to induce fragmentation of the calcific deposit and induce resorption. It has been shown in some studies to be better than sham treatment, but there is inconclusive evidence of its effectiveness.
- Surgery: chronic pain in the presence of calcific deposits that has failed to respond to conservative measures may be treated surgically. The majority of surgeons focus on the calcific deposit, which

can be identified at arthroscopy. The deposit can be decompressed and suctioned. Surgeons vary in their enthusiasm for also performing a sub-acromial decompression. Success rates for surgical decompression are in the region of 92% by 6 months.

Long head of biceps disorders

Causes

The biceps proximally comprises the long and short head tendons. The short head is a very short and muscular attachment to the coracoid. It is extra-articular and very rarely injured. However, the long head of biceps (LHB) is a long, 'ropy' tendon that follows a tortuous route from the superior glenoid, via the glenohumeral joint to the biceps muscle. It passes through a narrow biceps groove in the proximal humerus, where it is potentially unstable and contained by the biceps pulley mechanism. The biceps pulley is a confluence of the rotator cuff tendons and glenohumeral ligaments. Therefore injury to the rotator cuff can lead to biceps instability and inflammation. The LHB is also prone to high forces and has a poor vascularity, predisposing it to pathology. It also has a rich supply of sensory nerves, so is a powerful pain generator when affected.

The common disorders of the LHB are listed below.

- Biceps tendonitis: inflammation or degeneration of the LHB in the biceps groove from osteophytes or rotator cuff disease (Figure 4.6a).
- Biceps instability: medial subluxation of the LHB out of the groove with rotation of shoulder due to loss of the LHB stabilizers, the biceps pulley and rotator cuff (Figure 4.6b).
- Rupture: degenerative or traumatic rupture of the LHB tendon (Figure 4.6c).

History and examination

Biceps disease is commonly associated with rotator cuff tears, particularly of the subscapularis tendon. Therefore, the history will be similar to rotator cuff disease. Pain from the LHB is quite localized to the biceps groove and radiates down the biceps muscle. If there is instability of the tendon then painful clicking can be felt on rotating the shoulder.

A ruptured LHB can often create a deformity, known as the 'Popeye sign', where the biceps muscle tends to bunch up and appear more prominent. This is usually asymptomatic and only rarely is associated with cramping and some weakness in people who do heavy manual work.

The most useful clinical tests for LHB pain are:

- Speed's test: resisted flexion, with the shoulder flexed and elbow extended (Figure 4.7),
- direct tenderness over the biceps groove.

Investigations

Ultrasound scan is the most useful imaging for evaluating the LHB. It is easy to see fluid in the biceps sheath with biceps tendonitis and a subluxing or dislocated LHB is clearly seen with dynamic screening. Associated rotator cuff tears can also be seen.

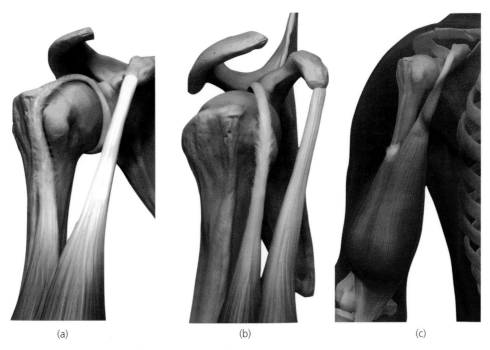

Figure 4.6 Biceps pathologies. (a) Biceps tendonitis. (b) Biceps instability. (c) Rupture.

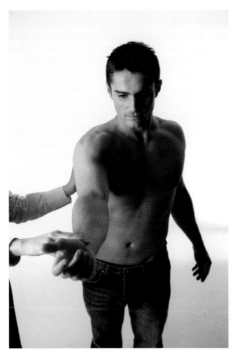

Figure 4.7 Speed's test.

Treatment

Physiotherapy to improve shoulder posture and the rotator cuff can relieve pressure on the LHB. Ultrasound guided injections into the LHB sheath can reduce inflammation. Corticosteroids can be used for this, but they can cause damage to the tendon proteins and weaken it. Hyaluronan injections are less likely to cause tendon weakness, but are less powerful than corticosteroids.

Surgical treatment of LHB pathologies is in the form of either *biceps tenotomy* or *tenodesis*. Tenotomy is division of the LHB near its insertion onto the glenoid and is a simple and quick method of pain relief. There is a risk of a Popeye sign. A tenodesis involves reattachment of the LHB to the proximal humerus bone or neighbouring tendons. Tenodesis reduces the risk of a Popeye sign, but can lead to pain at the tenodesis site in a small proportion of patients and is associated with a longer recovery period. Tenodesis is generally performed for young, lean and athletic individuals and tenotomy for older, less active people.

Further reading

Auplish S, Funk L. Rotator cuff tears in athletes. *Br J Hosp Med* 2009;**70**(**5**):234–238.

Beaudreuila J, Dhénainb M, Coudanec H, Mlika-Cabanneb N. Clinical practice guidelines for the surgical management of rotator cuff tears in adults. *Orthop Traumatol Surg Res* 2010;**96**:175–179.

Brox JI, Staf PH, Ljunggren AE, Brevik JI. Arthroscopic surgery compared with supervised exercises in patients with rotator cuff disease(stage I impingement syndrome). *BMJ* 1993;**307**:899–902.

Ejnisman B, Monteiro GC, Andreoli CV. Disorder of the long head of the biceps tendon. *Br J Sports Med* 2010;**44**:347–354.

Ellman H, Kay SP. Arthroscopic subacromial decompression for chronic impingement. Two to five-year results. *J Bone Joint Surg Br* 1991;**73**:395–398.

Funk L. shoulderdoc.co.uk (updated 22 April 2014).

Goutallier D, Postel JM, Bernageau J *et al.* Fatty muscle degeneration in cuff ruptures. Pre- and postoperative evaluation by CT scan. *Clin Orthop Relat Res* 1994;**304**:78–83.

Holmgren T, Björnsson Hallgren H, Öberg B *et al.* Effect of specific exercise strategy on need for surgery in patients with subacromial impingement syndrome: randomised controlled study. *BMJ* 2012;**344**:e787.

Lam F, Bhatia D, van Rooyen K, de Beer JF. Modern management of calcifying tendinitis of the shoulder. *Curr Orthop* 2006;**20**:446–452.

Moravek JE, Budge MD, Wiater JM. Current concepts in subacromial impingement and the role of acromioplasty. *Shoulder Elbow* 2012;**4**:244–254.

Nicholson GP, Goodman DA, Flatow EL, Bigliani LU. The acromion: morphologic condition and age-related changes. A study of 420 scapulas. *J Shoulder Elbow Surg* 1996;**5**(**1**):1–11.

Serafini G, Sconfienza LM, Lacelli F *et al.* Rotator cuff calcific tendonitis: short-term and 10-year outcomes after two-needle US-guided percutaneous treatment— nonrandomized controlled trial. *Radiology* 2009;**252**(**1**):157–164.

Simank HG, Dauer G, Schneider S, Loew M. Incidence of rotator cuff tears in shoulder dislocations and results of therapy in older patients. *Arch Orthop Trauma Surg* 2006;**126**(**4**):235–240.

CHAPTER 5

Shoulder: The Articular Structures

Lennard Funk

Wrightington, Wigan & Leigh NHS Trust, Wrightington, UK

OVERVIEW

- Labral injuries are common in sporting shoulder injuries.
- The best imaging is a magnetic resonance arthrogram, but it is not 100% accurate.
- Arthroscopy is the best diagnostic tool, which also allows direct repair.
- The muscles supply 60% of shoulder stability.
- Traumatic shoulder instability usually requires surgery, but motor control instability requires specialist rehabilitation.
- A normal glenohumeral joint radiograph is necessary to eliminate osteoarthritis and confirm the diagnosis of 'frozen shoulder'.
- Good-quality nerve conduction studies are needed to differentiate between an isolated nerve palsy and a neuralgic amyotrophy.
- Surgery is beneficial for an isolated nerve palsy, but not for neuralgic amyotrophy.

Introduction

In the previous chapter we considered the *sub-acromial* structures as potential sources of pain and dysfunction. We will now focus on the *articular* structures (including the articular labrum, biceps and capsule), which have a major impact on shoulder function and where injury can cause instability and impingement problems.

Labral injuries

Causes

The glenoid labrum (Figure 5.1) is a thickened fibrous band surrounding the glenoid cavity that provides stability to the glenohumeral joint. The labrum is frequently injured with sports injuries in young people, particularly with shoulder dislocations. The mechanism of injury determines the area of labral injury. The anterosuperior section of the labrum's attachment is looser and this extra 'give' makes injury less likely than the other areas where the labrum is very well attached.

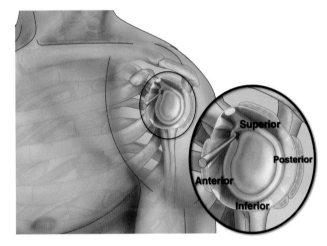

Figure 5.1 Glenoid labrum, showing the superior, anterior, posterior and inferior regions, with a hook demonstrating the loose anterosuperior region.

History and examination

Labral injuries are commonly sports-related. Large traumatic tears occur in contact sports with traumatic subluxations or dislocations of the shoulder. Repetitive, overhead sports lead to chronic tears of the labrum, usually at the superior labrum, and these injuries are known as superior labral anteroposterior (SLAP) tears (Figure 5.2).

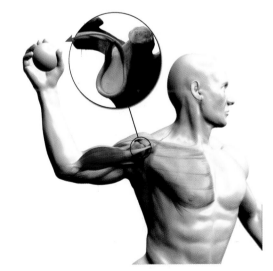

Figure 5.2 SLAP tear with overhead sport – the superior labrum is wrenched and twisted from it's attachment to the superior glenoid.

ABC of Common Soft Tissue Disorders, First Edition.
Edited by Francis Morris, Jim Wardrope and Paul Hattam.

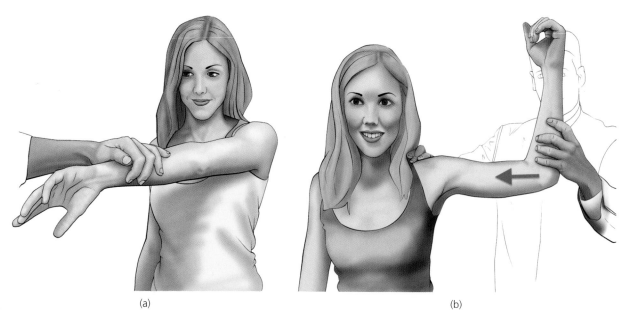

(a)   (b)

Figure 5.3 (a) O'Brien's test for SLAP tears. (b) Kibler's clunk test for labral tears. Green arrows, examiner's force; red arrows, patient's resistance.

Symptoms of a labral tear usually include:

- pain performing sport, such as throwing, overhead racquet sport and resistance exercises in the gym; the pain is typically felt on release of the ball, making contact between the ball and racquet and pushing exercises,
- painful clicking with activities,
- feelings of instability towards end range of movements, such as in full abduction and external rotation,
- loss of confidence in shoulder,
- dead arm symptoms or numbness or tingling towards end range of movements, such as in full abduction and external rotation.

Clinical examination tests are not sensitive and often non-specific, but some useful tests are outlined here.

- O'Brien's test for SLAP tears: pain is felt in the shoulder with resisted flexion when the arm is in full adduction and internal rotation. Pain is less when reproducing the resisted flexion with the arm in full external rotation (see Figure 5.3a).
- Kibler's clunk/crank test: the shoulder is loaded in the axial direction while it is rotated by the examiner (similar to the McMurray's test in the knee). A positive test is pain or clicking (Figure 5.3b).

Investigations

The most accurate investigation for labral tears is a shoulder arthroscopy, where the tear can be both seen and palpated with a probe. However, this is a surgical procedure. Therefore, less invasive techniques include plain magnetic resonance imaging (MRI) scans or an MR arthrogram (MRA).

Treatment

Most labral tears require surgical repair if sporting activities are significantly affected. A trial of physiotherapy is beneficial, as some patients will develop enough protective muscle strength and stability to return to sport. The time of the sporting season will also affect treatment decisions, as an athlete with a mid-season small labral tear may be able to continue playing and undergo repair at the end of season.

Shoulder instability

Shoulder dislocations and instability are common due to the inherent reliance on the soft tissues to stabilize the glenohumeral joint. Stability is provided by the dynamic (muscular) stabilizers and the static stabilizers.

Dynamic stabilizers:

- rotator cuff muscles: centralize and contain the humeral head against the glenoid,
- large movement muscles (create power and torque): deltoid, pectoralis major, latissimus dorsi and teres major,
- scapula muscles (provide a solid foundation for shoulder motion): rhomboids, trapezius serratus anterior and latissimus dorsi.

Static stabilizers:

- glenoid labrum: creates a chuck-block effect to contain the humeral head on the glenoid,
- glenohumeral ligaments: the glenohumeral joint capsule folds in complex ways to create thickened folds that correspondingly tighten and loosen in the extremes of range to contain the humeral head; the capsule also has proprioceptive nerve endings that activate the dynamic stabilizers in these positions,
- bones and joint: the shape and directions of the humeral head and glenoid affect stability; for example, a retroverted glenoid can predispose to posterior instability.

About 60% of shoulder stability is due to the muscular elements, with 40% coming from the static stabilizers, which highlights the importance of muscular rehabilitation in the treatment of shoulder stability.

Causes

There are three main types of shoulder instability, and it is essential to recognize this, as the type of instability determines the management.

Traumatic instability

Dislocations or subluxations with significant force are 'traumatic' and are commonly due to contact sports or significant injury to the shoulder. The initial dislocation usually requires manual relocation. Due to the amount of force that is associated with such an injury significant damage to the static stabilizers is common. These include:

- labral tears
- capsular stretching and sometimes a capsular tear (humeral avulsion of glenohumeral ligaments, HAGL)
- bony injuries, such as:
  - Hill–Sachs impaction injury to the humeral head,
  - bony fractures of the glenoid (e.g. bony Bankart lesion),
- osteochondral injuries,
- rotator cuff tears.

Atraumatic instability

The shoulder dislocates with minimal force, such as reaching up for an object or turning over in bed. Usually it will 'pop' back in itself or with a little help. Normally this type of dislocation does not need manual relocation. Subluxations can occur frequently and associated with certain positions, such as reaching overhead. This type of instability is associated joint hyper-laxity, such as the gymnast who over exerts. Common pathologies include small labral tears and abrasions, and over-stretching of the joint capsule with loss of proprioception. Secondary muscular instability ensues with progressive shoulder instability.

Motor-control instability

Some individuals can dislocate their shoulders without any history of trauma. Some may have started out dislocating their shoulder as a party trick; others may have always had shoulders that just 'fall' out of joint. This type of dislocation is usually painless and can be relocated easily. Both shoulders are commonly involved. The cause of this type of dislocation is usually a result of 'abnormal muscle patterning'. The strong muscles around the shoulder joint become dyssynchronous, causing them to pull the shoulder out of joint with active movement in a particular direction.

History

Shoulder instability is more common in younger people, usually from the mid-teens to the fourth decade. It is unusual in older groups. In older patients, shoulder dislocation may be associated with a rotator cuff tear.

The type of shoulder instability can be determined from the history, taking particular note of reported episodes of dislocations or subluxations. Sometimes patients may not report true dislocations or subluxations but may complain of 'a dead arm' or 'numbness' with the arm in extreme positions, loss of confidence in their shoulder, clicking, avoidance and apprehension with certain activities.

Examination

Clinical examination should include the labral tests (see the earlier section on Labral injuries), as well as assessment of shoulder instability and laxity and generalized ligamentous laxity.

Instability tests

- Anterior apprehension with Jobe's relocation test: with the patient sitting or supine the shoulder is gradually taken into abduction and external rotation. The patient will report apprehension at a certain point ('anterior apprehension'). At this point the examiner's puts gentle posterior pressure over the front of the shoulder joint. The patient then reports less apprehension ('Jobe's relocation positive'). See Figure 5.4a.
- Posterior apprehension test: the shoulder is positioned in maximal internal rotation and flexion, then loaded with a posteriorly directed force (see Figure 5.4b).
- Modified O'Brien's test for posterior instability: the shoulder is positioned in maximal internal rotation and flexion. The patient is asked to resist downward pressure on the forearm. Weakness (not pain) in this position is indicative of posterior instability (see Figure 5.4c).
- Apprehension sulcus test: with the patient seated or standing, gentle longitudinal downward traction is applied. Apprehension is a positive sign for inferior instability (see Figure 5.4d).

Investigations

Investigations are identical to labral injury investigations (see the section on Labral injuries). In older patients, an ultrasound scan may be appropriate as rotator cuff tears are more common.

Treatment

Acute traumatic shoulder dislocations must always be relocated as soon as possible. It is essential to assess the neurovascular status of the arm before and after relocation: specifically, the axillary nerve.

Management of shoulder instability depends on the type of instability, as described below.

- Traumatic instability: generally surgical repair is required for major structural lesions, as the recurrence rate with non-operative management is very high in young, active athletes. In non-athletic patients, non-operative treatment is an option depending on the severity of the structural lesions (i.e. large bony lesions have much higher risks of recurrent instability than smaller labral lesions). Therefore, the decisions should be made based on the functional demands and age of the patient as well as the severity of the pathological lesions found on MRA or computed tomography (CT) arthrogram.

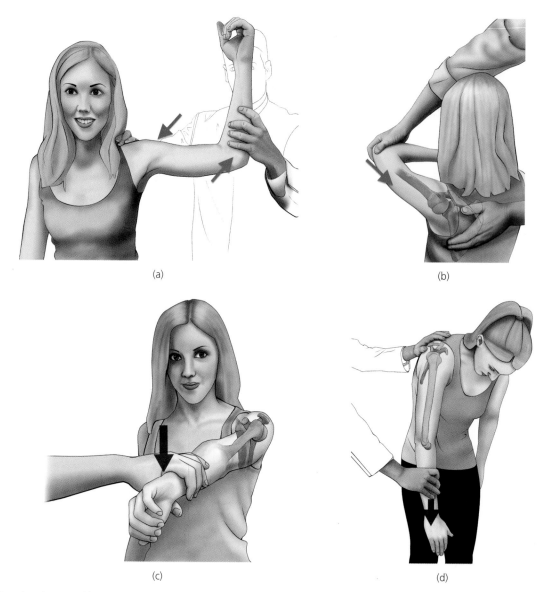

Figure 5.4 Apprehension tests. (a) Anterior. (b) Posterior. (c) Modified O'Brien's. (d) Anteroinferior sulcus. Green arrows, examiner's force.

- Atraumatic instability: most patients should improve with a proprioceptive, scapula and strengthening rehabilitation programme. This is best undertaken by an experienced phys-iotherapist who has been trained in shoulder rehabilitation, as incorrect rehabilitation can exacerbate the instability. If the shoulder laxity and proprioception are not improving with rehabilitation then a capsular plication procedure is often beneficial to stabilize the shoulder and aide the rehabilitation process.
- Motor-control instability: although this is rare, it is essential to clearly identify this group of patients from the atraumatic, hyperlax patients (which can be difficult). Surgery is frequently bound to fail and the mainstay of treatment is specialist shoulder rehabilitation, preferably within a multi-disciplinary shoulder unit.

Frozen shoulder

Causes

Frozen shoulder, also known as *adhesive capsulitis*, is a painful restriction of active and passive shoulder movements. Although the majority of patients presenting with frozen shoulder do not have an underlying cause (*primary frozen shoulder*), there is an increased incidence of this condition in patients with diabetes, Dupuytren's contracture, cardiac disease and stroke. *Secondary frozen shoulder* can occur after trauma, surgery or immobilization of the shoulder (Box 5.1).

Box 5.1 **Types of frozen shoulder**

Primary: associations

Diabetes
Dupuytren's contractures
Pulmonary pathologies
Thyroid pathologies
Breast cancer

Secondary

Post-traumatic
Post-operative
Post-immobilization

History and examination

The onset of primary frozen shoulder is typically spontaneous, although some patients may relate the onset of symptoms to a minor injury. Sudden onset and severe pain, particularly at night and aggravated by any movement of the shoulder, is a common presentation. The patient will exhibit stiffness of all movements, most notably passive restriction of external rotation. This is pathognomonic of the condition. Septic arthritis, acute calcific tendonitis and neuralgic amyotrophy are the main differential diagnoses in the early stages. Frozen shoulder is a diagnosis of exclusion. Along with suggestive clinical signs and symptoms, a normal radiograph is essential.

Natural history

Three classic phases of frozen shoulder are the 'freezing', 'frozen' and 'thawing' phases. The shoulder can pass through these phases fairly quickly within a few months, but in severe cases symptoms can persist for 2–3 years. Early recognition and appropriate intervention is key to achieving the fastest and most optimal resolution.

- Freezing phase: characterized by severe, unremitting pain of sudden onset. The pain can be so severe that patients present as an emergency. Typically there is a dull, constant throbbing pain at rest, with severe sharp pain on unguarded movements. As the pain gradually subsides stiffness sets in.
- Frozen phase: a painless and very stiff shoulder. Loss of external rotation is typical and present in almost all cases. Pain is only felt with unguarded and sudden movements.
- Thawing phase: movement and pain gradually resolve. Often, sub-acromial impingement symptoms persist due to weakness of the rotator cuff muscles.

Investigations

Normal plain radiographs of the glenohumeral joint are essential to diagnose a frozen shoulder. This excludes other conditions that can resemble a frozen shoulder, such as glenohumeral joint arthritis and calcific tendonitis. Ultrasound scans are also beneficial to exclude these, as well as demonstrating the rotator cuff in more detail.

Treatment

Treatment is proportionate to the severity and duration of symptoms. The first-line treatment includes a combination of oral analgesia, physiotherapy and glenohumeral joint corticosteroid injection(s). The focus in the earlier stages should be to reduce the inflammatory process and pain in order to permit mobilization of the shoulder, which will in turn reduce the loss of function and disability ensuing.

In the few cases where primary treatment fails, further intervention may be necessary in sufficiently symptomatic patients. Treatment choice is usually based on severity of disease, patient expectation and surgeon preference. The options are as follows.

- Arthrographic distension (hydrodilatation): injection of high-volume saline and long-acting corticosteroid is performed under radiographic guidance. This procedure is particularly appealing as it can be performed as an outpatient procedure, with low risk and high success rates.
- Manipulation under anaesthesia (MUA): a surgical procedure where the capsular adhesions are ruptured by controlled forceful manipulation of the shoulder under general anaesthesia. A corticosteroid injection is often also used. Although the risks are low, care needs to be exercised in osteoporotic bones and post-fracture cases.
- Arthroscopic capsular release: involves division of the contracted capsule under direct arthroscopic vision and has become very popular in modern shoulder practice due to the low risk of iatrogenic injury and improved pain relief and function. Success rates are over 95%, but recovery can take 3–6 months.

Neuralgic amyotrophy

Causes

Neuralgic amyotrophy is an uncommon condition affecting the shoulder and upper arm. The exact cause is not known. It is thought to be viral or autoimmune. It is known by numerous different names, such as Parsonage–Turner syndrome and brachial neuritis.

History and examination

It tends to affect young, active males primarily. The typical history is sudden pain followed by marked muscle weakness and wasting of the shoulder girdle and upper arm. Pain starts suddenly across the top of the shoulder blade and lasts from a few hours to a fortnight. The degree of pain may be variable and some patients don't recall a significant painful episode.

Then, a weakness of some of the muscles of the shoulder girdle and often of the arm develops. When the weakness appears, the pain usually stops. There is usually no loss of sensation associated with the weakness.

It may give rise to secondary shoulder impingement due to the muscle imbalance. Patients also develop a fatigue of the shoulder, particularly with overhead activities. In the acute phase the condition may resemble an acute frozen shoulder, calcific tendonitis or arthritis. In the chronic, weak phase it often resembles rotator cuff tears of the shoulder or nerve root compression.

Investigations

Nerve conduction studies (electromyography, EMG) and imaging studies are useful in establishing the diagnosis and assessing the amount of nerve degeneration and recovery. It is essential that all periscapular muscles are tested by an experienced neurophysiologist.

Treatment

No specific treatment has yet been proved efficient in neuralgic amyotrophy. In the early stages, pain may require treatment. Common painkillers are usually sufficient.

As pain subsides, physiotherapy is recommended. Passive range-of-motion exercises of the shoulder and elbow are suggested to maintain full range of motion. Active rehabilitation is undertaken only when some recovery of the affected muscle(s) is already obtained. Furthermore, all the upper body muscles should undergo rehabilitative exercises, and not only those presenting clinical weakness. It is also recommended that strength recovery reaches a plateau before the patient returns to sport.

The prognosis is generally good, since recovery of strength and sensation usually begins spontaneously, as early as 1 month after symptom onset, with about 75% recovery within 2 years. However, the period of time for complete recovery is very variable, ranging from 6 months to 5 years. It seems that the delay in recovering strength depends on the severity and duration of pain, weakness or both.

Suprascapular nerve palsy

Causes

The suprascapular nerve provides power to the supraspinatus and infraspinatus rotator cuff muscles. It is therefore an important nerve for shoulder function. It also provides 70% of the sensation from the deep shoulder joint.

The nerve follows a tortuous route from the brachial plexus, passing through the suprascapular notch under the transverse ligament of the scapula and then around the spine of the scapula in the spinoglenoid notch adjacent to the superior glenoid labrum (Figure 5.5). It is at the suprascapular notch and the spinoglenoid notch that it is prone to traction injury and compression from adjacent structures.

The common causes of suprascapular nerve injury are:

- compression from the transverse ligament in the suprascapular notch,
- ganglion paralabral cysts from labral tears,
- traction injuries,

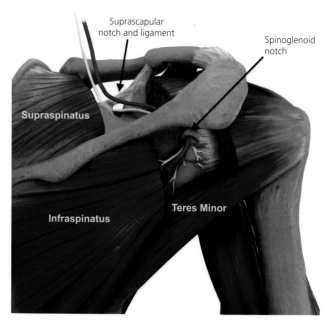

Figure 5.5 Route of the suprascapular nerve in the shoulder.

- iatrogenic pain as a surgical complication,
- neuritis: as part of neuralgic amyotrophy or isolated.

History and examination

The wasting and weakness of the muscles can be dramatic and rapid in their onset. If the nerve is affected at the suprascapular notch both supraspinatus and infraspinatus are affected, but if it is injured at the spinoglenoid notch then only the infraspinatus is affected.

Investigations

MRI scan can show paralabral ganglion cysts and neurogenic oedema with wasting of the affected muscles. Nerve conduction studies and EMG studies are predominantly diagnostic and can further clarify the area of injury.

Treatment

Treatment usually involves physiotherapy, with specific reactivation exercises and a scapula-control regimen. Avoidance of worsening activities should be observed to give the nerve time to recover without further aggravation or stretching. Surgery may be needed, especially if the cause of the problem is entrapment or compression. Surgical decompression of the nerve can be performed either endoscopically or with open surgery.

Further reading

Burkhart SS, Morgan CD. The peel-back mechanism: its role in producing and extending posterior type II SLAP lesions and its effect on SLAP repair rehabilitation. *Arthroscopy* 1998;**14**(**6**):637–640.

Chambler AFW, Carr AJ. The role of surgery in frozen shoulder. *J Bone Joint Surg Br* 2003;**85-B**:789–795.

Cummins CA, Messer TM, Nuber GW. Suprascapular nerve entrapment. *J Bone Joint Surg Br* 2000;**82-A**(**3**):415–424.

Fraser-Moodie JA, Shortt NL, Robinson CM. Injuries to the acromioclavicular joint. *J Bone Joint Surg Br* 2008;**90-B**:697–707.

Funk L, Snow M. SLAP tears of the glenoid labrum in contact athletes. *Clin J Sport Med* 2007;**17**(**1**):1–4.

Lafosse L, Tomasi A, Corbett S *et al.* Arthroscopic release of suprascapular nerve entrapment at the suprascapular notch: technique and preliminary results. *Arthroscopy* 2007;**23**(**1**):34–42.

Lewis A, Kitamura T, Bayley JIL. The classification of shoulder instability: new light through old windows. *Curr Orthop* 2004;**18**:97–108.

Malone AA, Funk L, Mohammed K, Ball C. Shoulder instability in the collision athlete - the collision shoulder. *Bone Joint Surg Br Proc* 2009;**91-B**:259.

Mazzocca AD, Arciero RA, Bicos J. Evaluation and treatment of acromioclavicular joint injuries. *Am J Sports Med* 2007;**35**:316.

Miller MD, Wirth MA, Rockwood CA. Thawing the frozen shoulder: the 'patient' patient. *Orthopedics* 1996;**19**:849–853.

Ng CY, Smith E, Funk L. Reliability of the traditional classification systems for acromioclavicular joint injuries by radiography. *Shoulder Elbow J* 2012;**4**(**4**):266–269.

Robinson CM, Jenkins PJ, White TO *et al.* Primary arthroscopic stabilization for a first-time anterior dislocation of the shoulder. A randomized, double-blind trial. *J Bone Joint Surg Am* 2008;**90**:708–721.

Safran MR. Nerve injury about the shoulder in athletes. *Am J Sports Med* 2004;**32**:1063–1074.

Sathasivam S, Lecky B, Manohar R, Selvan A. Neuralgic amyotrophy. *J Bone Joint Surg Br* 2008;**90-B**:550–553.

Shaffer B, Tibone JE, Kerlan RK. Frozen shoulder. *J Bone Joint Surg Am* 1992;**74**:738–746.

Smith C, Funk L. The glenoid labrum. *Shoulder Elbow J* 2010;**2**(**2**):87–93.

van Alfen N, van Engelen BGM. The clinical spectrum of neuralgic amyotrophy in 246 cases. *Brain* 2006;**129**:438–450.

Wang VW, Flatow E. Pathomechanics of acquired shoulder instability: a basic science perspective. *J Shoulder Elbow Surg* 2005;**14**:2S–11S.

Watson L, Bialocerkowski A, Dalziel R *et al.* Hydrodilatation (distension arthrography): a long-term clinical outcome series. *Br J Sports Med* 2007;**41**:167–173.

CHAPTER 6

Elbow

David Stanley[1] and Santosh Venkatachalam[2]

[1]Shoulder and Elbow Unit, Northern General Hospital, Sheffield Teaching Hospitals NHS Foundation Trust, Sheffield, UK
[2]Northumbria Healthcare, North Tyneside General Hospital, North Shields, UK

OVERVIEW

- This chapter introduces the common soft tissue disorders around the elbow.
- It identifies common presenting factors including patient demographics.
- The clinical signs to diagnose each condition are demonstrated.
- Recommendations are given for further imaging following clinical examination.
- Common treatment modalities of these conditions are discussed.

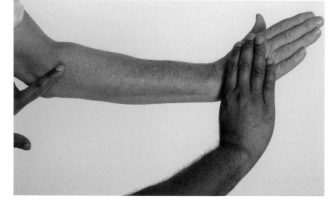

Figure 6.1 Provocative test for lateral epicondylitis (tennis elbow).

Lateral epicondylitis (tennis elbow)

Introduction

This condition occurs due to degenerative change, usually in the extensor origin (extensor carpis radialis brevis, extensor digitorum, extensor digiti minimi and extensor carpi ulnaris) at the lateral epicondylar region of the elbow. It is believed to result from repetitive wrist extension against resistance.

Epidemiology

The condition affects both men and women usually between the ages of 35 and 55 years. Although symptoms most commonly last from 6 to 24 months they can be persistent, with up to 20% of patients having long-term lateral elbow pain. The dominant arm is affected in around 75%.

Tennis elbow occurs in all types of occupation and sporting activity but is particularly likely in those that involve repetitive wrist extension like plumbing, painting, decorating, gardening, keyboard user, bricklaying and racquet sports.

Clinical features

The patient presents with an insidious onset of lateral elbow pain. The diagnosis is usually made clinically with tenderness at the lateral epicondylar area and pain on resisted extension of the wrist

(Figure 6.1). Resisted extension of the middle finger can also reproduce the symptoms. In patients who have had previous steroid injections an area of skin depigmentation and subcutaneous fat necrosis may be noted laterally at the epicondylar region.

Differential diagnoses

Differential diagnoses include lateral elbow instability (usually of traumatic origin), radiocapitellar arthritis (pain worse on resisted pronation and supination while the examiner holds the elbow flexed at 90° with palpation of the radial head), radial tunnel syndrome (pain localized distal to the lateral epicondyle area), and referred pain from the cervical spine and shoulder should all be considered in the differential diagnosis.

Treatment

The mainstay of management is patient education about the self-limiting nature of the condition. The majority of patients note that their symptoms settle down within a period of approximately 1 year. Activity modification to avoid repetitive twisting motions or high gripping forces can also be beneficial.

Currently, there is no favoured evidence-based treatment for tennis elbow. Options include oral/topical analgesics, use of elbow splints, topical heat/cold, rest and physiotherapy in the form of eccentric exercises. If these measures fail, the next step traditionally has been to inject steroids into the lateral epicondyle area. In the

ABC of Common Soft Tissue Disorders, First Edition.
Edited by Francis Morris, Jim Wardrope and Paul Hattam.
© 2016 John Wiley & Sons, Ltd. Published 2016 by John Wiley & Sons, Ltd.

long-term, however, this has not been found to be beneficial and may be harmful due to a higher rate of recurrence/tendon damage. More recently platelet-rich plasma (PRP) has been shown to be effective in a number of randomized control trials.

Surgery is generally considered as a last resort in those with tennis elbow resistant to conservative measures.

Medial epicondylitis (golfer's elbow)

Introduction
This condition is similar to lateral epicondylitis. It is thought to be secondary to overuse with repetitive microtrauma resulting in degenerative changes in the common flexor origin.

Epidemiology
Usually patients are in their fourth or fifth decades. Male and female distribution is equal and around 75% of cases are affected in their dominant elbow. Occupations and sporting activities that involve repetitive overuse, such as carpentry and sports like javelin throwing, weightlifting and golf, can predispose to this condition.

Clinical features
The normal presentation is an insidious onset of pain over the medial epicondylar region which worsens on forearm pronation and wrist flexion. The diagnosis is reached by clinical examination when it reveals tenderness over the medial epicondyle. Pain can be reproduced by flexing the wrist against resistance (Figure 6.2). The ulnar nerve is in close proximity to the muscular origin and this can result in concomitant pathology. As such, patients with medial epicondylitis may also present with features of ulnar nerve irritation. Typically this involves pins and needles in the ring and little fingers but may also include weakness of the small muscles of the hand.

Differential diagnoses
Differential diagnoses include post-traumatic medial elbow instability (patients with this condition will have a history of trauma

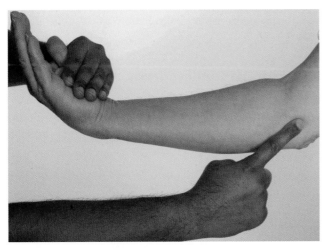

Figure 6.2 Provocative test for medial epicondylitis (golfer's elbow).

and features of elbow instability), cubital tunnel compression (sensory and motor ulnar nerve abnormalities) and elbow arthritis (restricted elbow range of movement and possible elbow locking due to loose bodies).

Treatment
The cornerstone of medial epicondylitis management is patient education and advice that the condition is normally self-limiting. Patients should however be warned that it may take many months to fully settle. It is appropriate to give a trial of conservative treatment with rest, analgesia and progressive physiotherapy rehabilitation. Particular attention should be given to throwing techniques and equipment design in athletes undertaking throwing activities in order to make the sporting procedure more ergonomic. Surgery is reserved for resistant golfer's elbow.

Pearls and pitfalls
Beware of patients who present with a sudden onset of elbow pain as this may indicate a traumatic avulsion of the common extensor/flexor origin. Symptoms in these patients are often similar to those with lateral and medial epicondylitis. Generally, if the patient can tell you the time and date of the injury, think of a traumatic cause. Epicondylitis of traumatic origin does not respond to non-operative measures and usually requires surgical intervention.

Olecranon bursitis (student's/miner's elbow)

Introduction
Olecranon bursitis occurs due to inflammation of the superficial bursa between the skin and the tip of the olecranon.

Epidemiology
The condition usually affects patients between 30 and 60 years of age. Around 65% of cases are non-infective in origin. Students and some forms of occupation that involve resting the elbow on hard surfaces can predispose to this condition due to repetitive trauma (hence the name student's or miner's elbow).

Clinical features
The normal presentation is a focal painful, red, fluctuant swelling, localized to the posterior aspect of the elbow. Terminal extension or flexion of the elbow may exacerbate the symptoms. Patients frequently give a history of recurrent similar symptoms. Although normally an isolated condition, occasionally it occurs in association with inflammatory arthropathy such as gout, rheumatoid arthritis or psoriatic arthritis.

Differential diagnosis
It is important to differentiate olecranon bursitis from septic arthritis of the elbow. In septic arthritis, all movements of the elbow are

painful and grossly restricted. Although the white cell count and inflammatory markers [C-reactive protein (CRP), erythrocyte sedimentation rate (ESR)] are usually raised in both conditions the levels are normally greater in septic arthritis. Radiographs may reveal calcification or gouty tophi or spur over the tip of the olecranon. The pain from triceps tendinitis is usually localized proximal to the olecranon tip. X-rays of the elbow generally reveal soft tissue swelling and or an incidental olecranon spur. Occasionally loose bodies in the bursa can be seen secondary to inflammatory arthropathy or pigmented villonodular synovitis (PVNS).

Treatment

Treatment with rest, ice, compression and elevation (RICE) and anti-inflammatory medications is usually effective. If there is no response to these interventions, aspiration of the bursa may be beneficial in relieving pain, confirming the diagnosis by microscopy culture/sensitivity and expediting recovery. Surgical excision of the bursa is indicated if the patient becomes systemically unwell or develops a resistant bursitis or recurrent problem.

Pearls and pitfalls

Aspiration should only be considered when non-invasive measures fail or infection is suspected. This is because aspiration carries a risk of infection and may convert a sterile bursitis into an infected one. In addition, it may also result in a chronic draining sinus tract.

Complete distal biceps rupture

Introduction

The biceps is the main supinator of the forearm and a flexor of the elbow.

Epidemiology

Complete ruptures of the distal biceps tendon comprise 3% of all biceps ruptures (proximal long head biceps rupture 97%). Ruptures occur most commonly in middle-aged men with sudden unanticipated eccentric loading of the biceps. Mechanisms of injury include sudden lifting of weights when the elbow is in mid-flexion or elbow flexion against a forceful elbow extension force, such as when attempting to catch a heavy falling object.

Clinical features

Patients present with a history of injury and pain over the front of the elbow. They may mention hearing a pop or experiencing a tearing feeling in the elbow followed by loss of biceps strength. If the injury has occurred more than 24 hours before presentation there is usually significant bruising over the anterior aspect of the elbow and forearm. The history should include enquiry regarding anabolic steroid abuse as these injuries are not infrequent in bodybuilders and gym users.

The diagnosis can normally be made clinically with proximal migration of the distal biceps and reduced supination strength

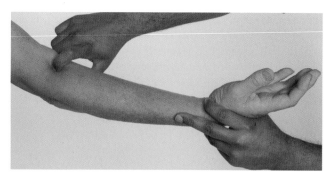

Figure 6.3 Hook test for checking distal biceps integrity.

when compared to the uninjured arm. In addition the patient will have a positive coat hanger/hook test. This test is performed by asking the patient to actively supinate the forearm with the elbow flexed to 90°. An intact biceps tendon allows the examiner to hook their index finger under the biceps tendon from the lateral side (Figure 6.3). When there is a distal biceps avulsion, the cord-like distal biceps tendon is absent and the examiner cannot hook a finger around the tendon.

Differential diagnosis

When there is doubt, an ultrasound scan or magnetic resonance imaging (MRI) with flexion, abduction and supination (FABS) views will confirm the diagnosis. Distal biceps ruptures result in loss of around 30–35% flexion strength and 40–55% supination strength.

Treatment

In low-demand patients surgical treatment may not always be required and the patient can make the decision taking into account the potential benefits of treatment and surgical risks. Surgical exploration and tendon repair, however, is the preferred management option particularly in those undertaking manual work and active individuals. It is important that the diagnosis is made in the early period after injury as the potential risks of surgery and difficulties in obtaining a satisfactory primary repair increase with time. Surgery is best performed within 2–3 weeks of the primary injury.

Distal biceps tendinopathy

Introduction

Patients with biceps tendinopathy present with pain around the front of the elbow which is worse on flexing or supinating the elbow against resistance.

Differential diagnosis

Radial tuberosity bursitis can mimic this condition. Further imaging with ultrasound or MRI can help confirm the diagnosis. MRI is more specific and sensitive in identifying tendinopathic changes or an inflamed bursa.

Treatment

Rest, patient education, anti-inflammatory drugs and modification of activities are the mainstay of treatment. An ultrasound-guided local steroid injection into the sheath/bursa may reduce inflammation but carries the risk of causing a tendon rupture if injected into the substance of the tendon.

Pearls and pitfalls

If the patient has typical history of biceps tendon rupture but the tendon can be palpated in the antecubital fossa, a partial rupture should be considered. The bicipital aponeurosis can remain intact and can be mistaken for an intact biceps tendon. Early diagnosis and treatment is essential, as with delayed presentation a primary repair may not be possible and reconstruction with a graft may be required.

Ulnar neuritis (cubital tunnel syndrome)

Introduction

This is one of the most common peripheral nerve entrapments encountered in clinical practice. It occurs due to compression of the ulnar nerve at the elbow as it passes behind the medial epicondyle.

Clinical features

Patients present with pain behind the elbow radiating pain down the inner aspect of the forearm. They complain of pins and needles along the ulnar nerve distribution most commonly affecting the little finger and the ulnar aspect of the ring finger. These symptoms may be exacerbated by prolonged elbow flexion such as holding a phone to the ear. Patients may also wake up in the night with pins and needles in their fingers.

Direct palpation of the nerve behind the medial epicondyle is sensitive (Figure 6.4) and Tinel's sign (tapping the nerve)

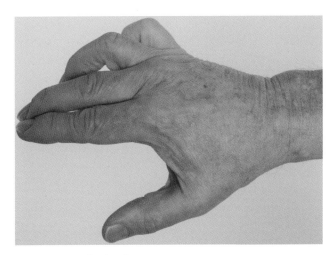

Figure 6.5 Ulnar claw hand.

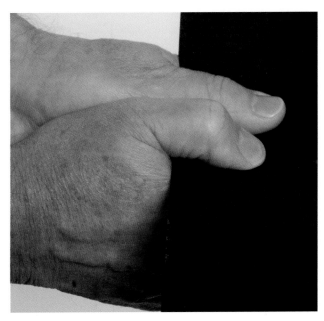

Figure 6.6 Froment's sign.

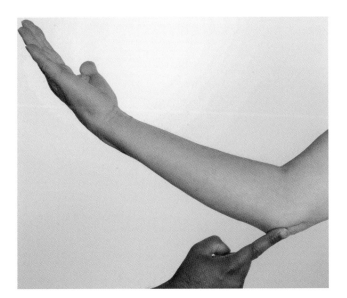

Figure 6.4 Palpation of ulnar nerve in the cubital tunnel posterior to the medial epicondyle.

reproduces the symptoms. Phalen's sign (hyperflexing the elbow for a period of approximately 1 minute) is also positive. In addition to sensory deficits motor function of the hand may be affected, resulting in clawing of the little and ring fingers (Figure 6.5) together with small-muscle wasting. Typical motor deficits include wasting of the first dorsal interosseous space, weakness of the abductors and adductors of the fingers and a positive Froment's sign (Figure 6.6; flexion of the interphalangeal joint of the thumb due to compensation by flexor pollicis longus for a weak adductor pollicis). The test is performed by asking the patient to hold a sheet of paper between the first web space against resistance. Wartenberg finger escape sign can be present with persistent abduction of the little finger (Figure 6.7). This is due to the weakness of the adductor of the little finger (palmar interossei), resulting in over-action of extensor digiti minimi, which is located eccentrically over the metacarpophalangeal joint.

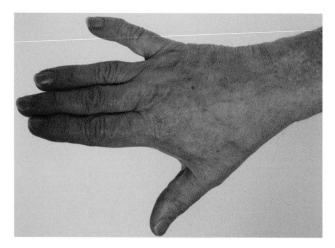

Figure 6.7 Wartenberg sign.

Differential diagnoses

These include golfer's elbow (location of pain in more anterior while the ulnar nerve is located posterior to medial epicondyle, Figure 6.4) and instability of the elbow joint. The cervical spine should always be assessed in case the neurological symptoms are due to more proximal nerve compression. Confirmation is based on nerve conduction studies, which reveal slowing of the conduction velocity within the ulnar nerve across the elbow.

Treatment

Conservative management involves advice to avoid elbow flexion for prolonged periods. However, if there are progressive sensory or motor deficits, surgical intervention is warranted.

Pearls and pitfalls

Beware of conditions that cause more proximal compression at the level of the cervical spine or brachial plexus. Conditions like Pancoast tumour and other causes of brachial plexopathy can mimic ulnar nerve neuropathy. Occasionally patients will have ulnar nerve compression at the elbow and a more proximal nerve compression (double crush phenomenon).

Further reading

Bisset L, Paungmali A, Vicenzio B *et al.* A systematic review and meta-analysis of clinical trials on physical interventions for lateral epicondylalgia. *Br J Sports Med* 2005;**39**(7):411–422.

Elhassan B, Steinmann SP. Entrapment neuropathy of the ulnar nerve. *J Am Acad Orthop Surg* 2007;**15**(11):672–681.

Lo My, Safran MR. Surgical treatment of lateral epicondylistis. A systematic review. *Clin Orthop* 2007;**463**:98–106.

O'Driscoll SW, Gonclaves LB, Dietz P. The hook test for distal biceps tendon avulsion. *Am J Sports Med* 2007;**35**(11):1865–1869.

Peerbooms JC, Sulimer J, Bruijn DJ *et al.* Effect of an autologous platelet concentrate in lateral epicondylitis, a double-blind randomized controlled trial: PRP versus corticosteroid injection with a 1 year follow up. *Am J Sports Med* 2010;**38**(2):255–262.

CHAPTER 7

Soft Tissue Disorders at the Wrist

David Knott

Dorset HealthCare University NHS Foundation Trust, Poole, UK

> **OVERVIEW**
> - The wrist is a compact area with many soft tissue structures prone to injury or overuse.
> - Diagnosis of most soft tissue disorders at the wrist is possible with a methodical history and examination.
> - Carpal tunnel syndrome is the commonest peripheral nerve entrapment syndrome.
> - de Quervain's tenosynovitis is easy to diagnose and usually treatable without the need for surgery.
> - The triangular fibrocartilage complex is prone to degeneration and injury and is a potential cause of ulnar-aspect wrist pain.

Basic anatomy

The wrist is a small body area but it contains a large number of tissues that can potentially cause pain. In addition to the distal radio-ulnar, radio-carpal and intercarpal joints there are many soft tissues: muscles, tendons, ligaments, nerves and a fibrocartilage disc. In this chapter we will consider the common soft tissue disorders occurring around the wrist.

History

The history should ideally follow a standard musculoskeletal approach such as that developed by the late James Cyriax. As the wrist is a superficial and distal limb joint, symptoms are usually well localized and it lends itself readily to examination and palpation. Diagnosis will usually be possible without the need for further investigations.

Key points are outlined here.

- Age and occupation/leisure activities: many soft tissue wrist problems arise as a result of overuse or trauma; in older age, degenerative problems arise although these are more commonly in the joints.

- Site and spread: wrist pain will normally be well localized with little spread; pain and neurological symptoms may be referred into the hand, however, and a more proximal source must be considered.
- Onset and duration: was it acute/traumatic – in which case think of fracture, sprains or triangular fibrocartilage complex (TFCC) injury – or gradual – in which case think more of tendon pathology or carpal tunnel syndrome?
- Behaviour/other symptoms: what makes it worse? Think of overuse/occupational factors. Ask about other symptoms, especially tingling, numbness or weakness in the hand.
- Past medical history: particularly other joint problems, conditions that could predispose to carpal tunnel syndrome (pregnancy, thyroid disease, diabetes etc.) and medication.

Examination

Examination of the wrist should include the following.

- Inspection: for any bony deformity (previous fractures etc.), colour changes such as redness or bruising, any muscle wasting (especially in the thenar and hypothenar muscles of the hand) and any swellings around the wrist (joint effusions, ganglia etc.).
- Passive movements: pronation and supination, passive flexion and extension, and radial and ulnar deviation. Although these movements mainly test the distal radio-ulnar and radio-carpal joints, adjacent soft tissues are also stretched and compressed and may elicit pain.
- Resisted testing: isometric (static) tests at the wrist of extension, flexion, radial and ulnar deviation and extension, flexion, abduction and adduction of the thumb isolate contractile (muscles, tendons and teno-osseous attachment) problems. Pain will commonly be reproduced on static contraction of the tissue.
- Palpation (for tenderness) along a particular tissue such as a tendon or joint line to more accurately localize pathology once a presumptive diagnosis has been made.
- Any additional or special tests that seem appropriate, such as Finklestein's test (see below, under de Quervain's tenosynovitis) or axial compression of the thumb for the trapeziometacarpal joint.

ABC of Common Soft Tissue Disorders, First Edition.
Edited by Francis Morris, Jim Wardrope and Paul Hattam.
© 2016 John Wiley & Sons, Ltd. Published 2016 by John Wiley & Sons, Ltd.

The most commonly encountered soft tissue disorders at the wrist are:

- carpal tunnel syndrome,
- de Quervain's tenosynovitis,
- intersection syndrome,
- triangular fibrocartilage complex (TFCC) pathology.

Carpal tunnel syndrome

Incidence

This is the commonest peripheral nerve entrapment syndrome with a crude incidence rate of approximately 1–3% in a general practice population with peak incidence in the age group 45–64 years. The condition is more common in women than men, with a ratio of 3:1.

Basic anatomy

The carpal tunnel is bounded dorsally by the arch of the carpal bones and ventrally by the flexor retinaculum. It allows for the transmission of the deep and superficial finger flexor tendons, the flexor pollicis longus tendon and the median nerve from the forearm into the hand. Clinically, the proximal extent of the carpal tunnel is marked by the distal wrist crease (running between the pisiform and the tubercle of the scaphoid bone). See Figure 7.1.

The median nerve usually runs in the midline of the wrist underneath the palmaris longus (if present) although individual variation in location can occur in the location of the main nerve and especially the motor branch. This can be of importance with injection and particularly with surgical decompression. See Figure 7.2.

Cause

The syndrome occurs when the relative pressure within the tunnel upon the median nerve is increased, as a result of either a reduced tunnel volume or an increase in the soft tissue volume in the tunnel. Symptoms will be aggravated when the median nerve is then subjected to more stress by wrist movement into flexion or extension, especially if sustained.

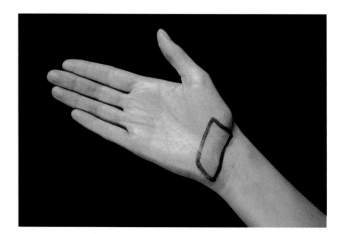

Figure 7.1 The extent of the flexor retinaculum which overlies the median nerve at the carpal tunnel, its most proximal border attaching to the pisiform and tubercle of the scaphoid bone.

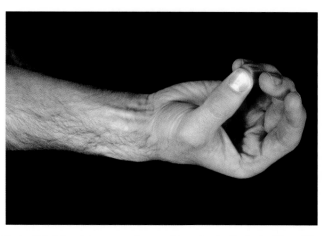

Figure 7.2 Palmaris longus can be a useful marker to site the position of the median nerve as it enters the carpal tunnel. If the patient opposes the thumb and fifth finger the tendon becomes evident. If it is absent, the crease between the thenar and hypothenar eminence denotes the nerve's position.

Many cases are idiopathic but certain underlying causes are also recognized, the more common being:

- pregnancy (especially later stages),
- hypothyroidism,
- diabetes mellitus,
- arthritis at the wrist,
- previous fracture at wrist with displacement/deformity.

Symptoms will include:

- paraesthesiae and/or numbness in the radial three or four digits: usually intermittent in milder cases and continuous in more severe cases,
- pain or discomfort in the palm (which may refer proximally up the arm),
- thenar muscle wasting and weakness in advanced cases,
- often being worse during the night and on waking.

Diagnosis

Diagnosis will include the history as above. Examination of the cervical spine may be necessary if the history is at all suggestive of cervical nerve root involvement or the distribution of paraesthesiae is inconsistent with the cutaneous supply of the medial nerve. Physical examination of the hand and wrist should include assessment of thenar muscles for any wasting/weakness and then provocation tests, the most common being the following three.

- Tinel's test: tapping over the mid-point of the carpal tunnel with a finger or percussion hammer produces temporary paraesthesiae in the median nerve distribution. Commonly used as a diagnostic aid (although studies show significant variability in terms of sensitivity and specificity; Hattam and Smeatham 2010) and also to help predict those patients who will recover well following decompressive surgery.
- Phalen's test: the wrist is held in full passive flexion for at least 1 minute. A positive test is the production of paraesthesiae in the median nerve distribution, and maybe also pain.

- Carpal compression test: firm pressure with the thumb over the mid-point of the carpal tunnel for up to 1 minute. Again, a positive test is the production of paraesthesiae and maybe pain. This is seen by many as a more sensitive test and is also useful in those patients who do not have full wrist flexion.

Although the history and examination will usually yield the correct diagnosis, in atypical presentations nerve conduction studies can be requested. Although these may be useful in the diagnosis of carpal tunnel syndrome and also in grading its severity, it must be remembered that there can be false negative and false positive results.

Treatment

- Correction of any underlying or predisposing conditions or activities if this is possible.
- Splinting of the wrist – traditionally during the night – to maintain the wrist in a position in which the median nerve is under minimum stress. Research suggests that the median nerve is least stressed in a neutral position although sometimes a small degree of extension is helpful (Weiss *et al.* 1995).
- Corticosteroid injection: a common and effective treatment that is widely used in practice. Success rates of 50–66% may be expected in the medium to long term (Shadel-Hopfner *et al.* 2001), with higher success rates in milder cases. Various techniques utilizing differing steroids in differing doses, and differing insertion points, have been described. Certainly, keeping the volume to a minimum is advisable with 0.5 ml of triamcinolone acetonide (40 mg/ml) sufficient. The use of local anaesthetic also leaves the patient with a numb hand for a couple of hours and is not recommended. The insertion point should be on the ulnar side of the palmaris longus tendon with the needle (25 mm, 25 gauge) being angled so that its tip ends up under the proximal part of the flexor retinaculum.
- Surgical decompression: this is the treatment of choice for more severe cases, especially for those with thenar muscle wasting, and for milder cases not responding to, or recurring after, splinting or injection. Recurrence after surgery is not impossible but is much less common than after injection.

de Quervain's tenosynovitis

Anatomy

In this condition, there is inflammation of the common sheath of the abductor pollicis longus (APL) and extensor pollicis brevis (EPB) tendons at or around the radial styloid process (see Figure 7.3).

Cause

de Quervain's tenosynovitis is usually an overuse-type injury although it can occasionally result from trauma. It tends to present sub-acutely or chronically with pain at the radial aspect of the wrist, made worse by activity. Repetitive work or leisure activities involving repeated thumb extension/abduction are the commonest cause.

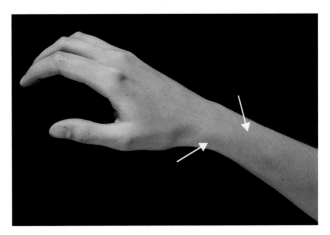

Figure 7.3 Lower left arrow: the site of de Quervain's tenosynovitis as the tendons of APL and EPB pass over the wrist joint. Upper right arrow: the site of intersection syndrome.

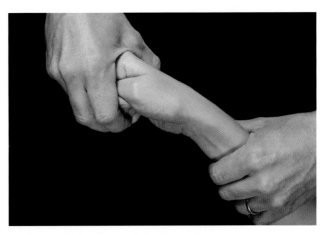

Figure 7.4 Finklestein's test: the thumb is positioned into the palm of the hand and fingers wrapped around. The wrist is then taken gently into ulnar deviation. This puts the tendons and sheath under tension and will reproduce the patient's symptoms.

Diagnosis

Diagnosis is almost always clinical (although, if in doubt, ultrasound scan will be helpful) and findings include:

- local tenderness of the ABL and EPB tendons near the radial styloid process,
- pain on resisted thumb extension and/or abduction,
- pain on passive thumb flexion, especially if wrist ulnar deviation is then added (Finklestein's test; Figure 7.4).

Treatment

- Corticosteroid injection: the most effective treatment is corticosteroid injection (10–20 mg of triamcinolone acetonide mixed with around 0.5 ml of local anaesthetic into the common tendon sheath) followed by rest and then activity modification to prevent recurrence. *Clinical tip*: given the superficial nature of the injection site, some practitioners may prefer to use hydrocortisone as there will be less risk of inadvertent soft tissue atrophy and depigmentation if the injection is misplaced external to the sheath.

- Physiotherapy and splinting could be used as an alternative if injection is not possible, unwanted or contraindicated. *Clinical tip*: occasionally, the condition fails to settle or keeps recurring which may be due to an abnormality of the sheath causing stenosis. Anatomical variants where each tendon has its own sheath have been observed, which may influence treatment outcome. These cases may well need a surgical decompression of the tendon sheath.

Intersection syndrome (oarsman's wrist)

Anatomy
Less commonly, the same two tendons that are involved in de Quervain's (APL and EPB) can also be involved in intersection syndrome. The tendons are involved more proximally in this case, at the point where they wind around the lower radius, crossing the tendons of extensor carpi radialis longus and brevis, which can cause friction between the two sets of tendons (see Figure 7.3).

Symptoms
This condition is less common than de Quervain's, and tends to present more acutely as a result of overuse. There is likely to be some redness, swelling and maybe crepitus, usually about 3 cm or so proximal to the radial styloid.

Treatment
It will often settle with rest, ice and anti-inflammatory (oral or topical) medication. However, if it does not, then it should respond to physiotherapy treatment. The tendons are not sheathed at this location and injection is not an effective option.

Triangular fibrocartilage complex (TFCC) pathology

Anatomy
The TFCC of the wrist sits in the lower radio-ulnar joint with attachments to the base of the ulnar styloid process and the edge of the radius just proximal to the radio-carpal articular surface. It serves to cover the head of the ulna, to increase the articular surface of the wrist joint and to transmit and absorb load, especially of a compressive nature, at the wrist. It is also a stabilizer of the lower radio-ulnar joint.

Cause
Pathology occurs either as a result of trauma (falls, rotational strains) or degeneration. The latter is a common finding, being present in 30–70% of cadavers, but is often asymptomatic. Degeneration is more common in those wrists exhibiting positive ulnar variance (when the ulnar is relatively lengthened compared to the radius). It will also be more common in wrists subjected to repetitive trauma or strain such as in gymnasts or some musicians.

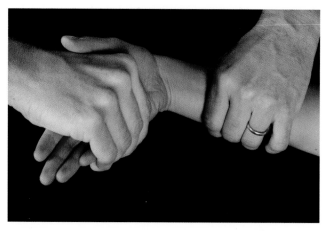

Figure 7.5 The TFCC test.

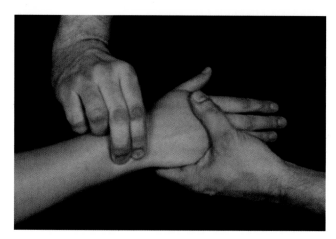

Figure 7.6 Piano key test.

Symptoms
Patients will normally present with pain at the ulnar aspect of the wrist, sometimes aching and sometimes sharp and stabbing. It will often be worse with certain activities. Patients may report clicking during movement.

Examination
Examination will usually reveal pain on one or more passive wrist movements (usually ulnar deviation), tenderness over the ulnar aspect of the wrist joint and a positive grind test (or ulnar meniscal compression test). A swelling is sometimes found in association with TFCC disorders.

Clinical tip
The TFCC compression test (Figure 7.5) is performed by taking the wrist through an arc of ulnar deviation passively while applying some axial compression.

Clinical tip
If there has been substantial trauma, concurrent injury of the inferior radio-ulnar joint can be assessed by using the piano key test

(Figure 7.6), which assesses instability of the joint. The patient sits with the forearm fully pronated and supported on a table. A downward pressure is applied to the distal end of the ulna, mimicking the action of pressing a piano key. Pain accompanied by excess movement and a more elastic end-feel denotes a positive result.

Investigations

Investigations could include plain x-ray – although this will not show the TFCC, it may demonstrate ulnar variance and any degenerative change in the joints – and magnetic resonance imaging (MRI) scan to demonstrate the TFCC itself.

Treatment

Analgesia, anti-inflammatory medication, splinting or corticosteroid injection can all be tried and may give relief. If symptoms persist, however, then surgery in the form of arthroscopy and debridement, or in some cases open surgery and TFCC repair, may be required.

Less common soft tissue disorders

Other soft tissues at the wrist can become painful, usually due to either trauma or overuse. These include the following.

- Collateral ligament sprain: either the ulnar or radial collateral ligaments may be injured. Presentation will normally include an appropriate history, localized pain and tenderness, and pain on passive stretch of the affected ligament. Treatment will usually be with physiotherapy but, in stubborn cases, a small amount of corticosteroid could be injected at a bony attachment.
- Scapholunate ligament injury: one of the more common ligament injuries at the wrist and a major factor for wrist instability and common wrist pain. Suspicion may be raised by a widened scapholunate joint space on plain x-ray. Clinically there may be a positive Watson's test (or scaphoid shift test, where the scaphoid is subluxed dorsally relative to the radius; Hattam and Smeatham 2010). MRI scan may demonstrate the lesion (although sensitivity is lower than ideal; Shadel-Hopfner et al. 2001) or else arthroscopy will be needed. If symptoms are sufficiently troublesome then surgical repair is indicated.
- Tendinopathy or tendinitis: any of the wrist and finger flexor or extensor tendons, or those of the thumb, can potentially become inflamed with overuse, be injured or develop a degenerative tendinopathy, although these are all less common than de Quervain's. Diagnosis should be possible through knowledge of wrist anatomy allied to a careful examination using the selective tension-type approach and palpation. Treatment will then usually be either physiotherapy or steroid injection although rest, ice, splinting and medication can all be tried first if desired.

Further reading

Atroshi I, Gummesson C, Johnsson R *et al.* Prevalence of carpal tunnel syndrome in a general population. *J Am Med Assoc* 1999;**282**(**2**):153–158.

Bongers FJM, Schellevis FG, van den Bosch WJHM, van der Zee J. Carpal tunnel syndrome in general practice (1987 and 2001): incidence and the role of occupational and non-occupational factors. *Br J Gen Pract* 2007;**57**(**534**):36–39.

Hattam P, Smeatham A. *Special tests in musculoskeletal examination: an evidence-based guide for clinicians.* Churchill Livingstone, London, 2010.

Mizia E, Klimek-Piotrowska W, Walocha J *et al.* The median nerve in the carpal tunnel. *Folia Morphol (Warsz)* 2011;**70**(**1**):41–46.

Shadel-Hopfner M, Iwinska-Zelder J, Braus T *et al.* MRI versus arthroscopy in the diagnosis of scapholunate ligament injury. *J Hand Surg Br* 2001;**26**(**1**):17–21.

Weiss ND, Gordon L, Bloom T *et al.* Position of the wrist associated with the lowest carpal-tunnel pressure: implications for splint design. *J Bone Joint Surg Am* 1995;**77**(**11**):1695–1699.

CHAPTER 8

Soft Tissue Injuries of the Hand

Helen Cugnoni

Homerton University Hospital, London, UK

OVERVIEW

- This chapter highlights the disproportionate impact even the most insignificant of hand injuries can have on a person's ability to carry out simple tasks.
- It outlines 'ALOHA' history: **a**ge of patient, **l**eisure activities, **o**ccupation, **h**and dominance, **a**ge of injury.
- The structures involved are tendons or ligaments.
- Conservative management with splints and/or physiotherapy is the mainstay of treatment.
- Appropriate follow-up is crucial.

Introduction

Anyone who has sustained even a 'minor' hand injury such as a mallet finger will know how much disability this will cause in everyday activity. The hand is a highly complex unit capable of a range of activities, from power lifting to fast complex precision movement. The sensory function of the hand is of major importance. Establish the 'ALOHA' history:

- **a**ge of patient: soft tissue hand injuries in children are usually well tolerated, recover in 2–3 weeks and have few sequelae; in older patients, apparently insignificant injuries may have a disproportionate effect on the ability to perform the activities of daily living,
- **l**eisure activities: sport, playing musical instruments and craftwork,
- **o**ccupation: the functional demands of a lumberjack and a professional musician will be quite different; also, many kitchen workers are not allowed to work while wearing any kind of hand dressing, resulting in potential loss of earnings or possible redundancy,
- **h**and dominance: often this is not recorded,
- **a**ge of injury: if there is any delay in presentation or initiation of treatment, time to recovery is longer and functional outcome is harder to predict.

On examination follow the normal 'look/feel/move' routine. In addition there are a number of specific tests of tendon function that need to be performed (see the flexor and extensor tendon sections) and sensation should be checked.

Tendon injuries at the distal interphalangeal joint (DIPJ)

Mallet finger: rupture of the extensor tendon at the DIPJ

This is the commonest tendon injury of the hand caused by either rupture of the extensor tendon at its insertion or an avulsion fracture involving the insertion of the terminal extensor tendon into the distal phalanx.

The patient presents with a flexion deformity at the DIPJ, often after fairly minor trauma that causes a forced flexion. Occasionally the tendon is divided by an open incised wound. It is easy to passively extend the joint but the distal phalanx will instantly droop into flexion when it is left unsupported. There is usually pain, tenderness and sometimes swelling.

Management

At the insertion into the base of the distal phalanx, the extensor tendon of the finger is a flat structure. In closed ruptures the divided ends are friable and frond-like, making surgical repair problematic. Management is usually conservative.

Plain radiography

This is done to establish whether or not there is an associated avulsion fracture fragment as this will result in improved healing and hence a more predictable functional outcome (Figure 8.1b). If the avulsion fragment involves more than one third of the articular surface the patient should be referred for internal fixation (Figure 8.1c).

Extension splint

Most mallet finger injuries are treated by immobilization of the DIPJ in extension, with an extension splint (Figure 8.2). The patient is given clear instructions that the splint must be worn continuously. The only time it should be removed is for washing; even then the

ABC of Common Soft Tissue Disorders, First Edition.
Edited by Francis Morris, Jim Wardrope and Paul Hattam.
© 2016 John Wiley & Sons, Ltd. Published 2016 by John Wiley & Sons, Ltd.

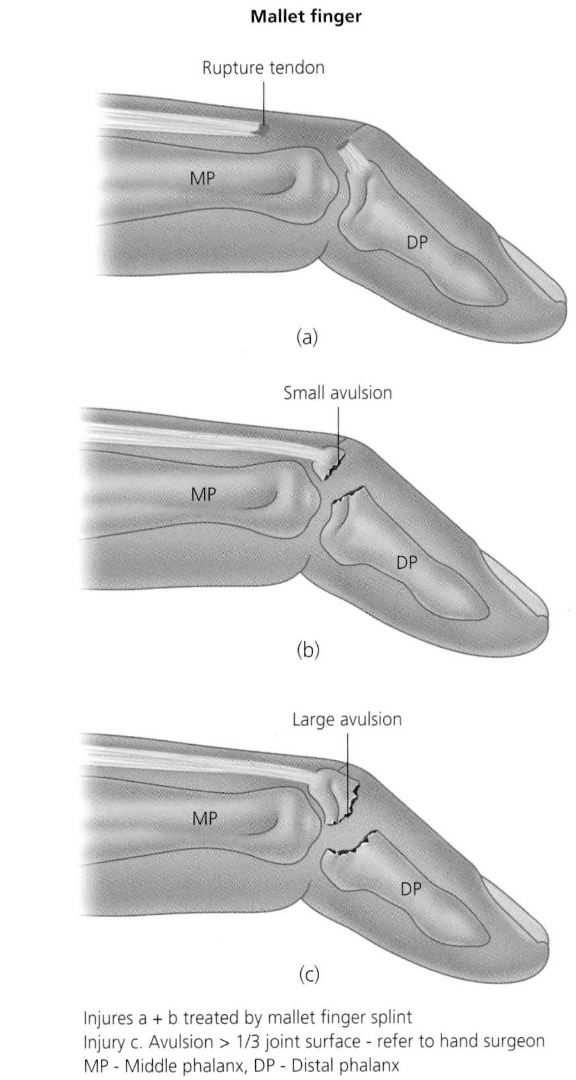

Mallet finger

Rupture tendon

(a)

Small avulsion

(b)

Large avulsion

(c)

Injures a + b treated by mallet finger splint
Injury c. Avulsion > 1/3 joint surface - refer to hand surgeon
MP - Middle phalanx, DP - Distal phalanx

Figure 8.1 Mallet finger.

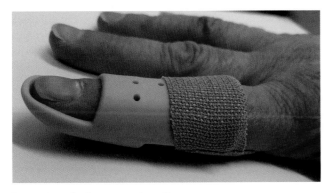

Figure 8.2 Mallet finger extension splint.

distal phalanx should be supported by the patient's other hand or on a flat surface.

Follow-up
The patient should be reviewed at 3 weeks to check progress and to ensure compliance with treatment. Most patients will need to stay in the splint for between 6 and 8 weeks, before gentle mobilization of the DIPJ.

Jersey finger: rupture of the flexor tendon at the DIPJ
Introduction
The flexor digitorum profundus (FDP) is partially or completely ruptured at its attachment to the distal phalanx, sometimes with a fragment of bone is avulsed from the base of the distal phalanx. The torn FDP tendon can retract towards the PIPJ or even into the palm of the hand. Affected patients lose the ability to actively flex at the DIPJ.

The term 'jersey finger' is used because the injury often occurs in rugby or American football players who have tried to make a tackle by grabbing an opponent's jersey/shirt. It is also an injury common to climbers who have taken their full body weight through a fingertip after a slip. This causes hyperextension at the DIPJ while the proximal portion of the finger is flexed. There is pain, tenderness, swelling and bruising over the volar aspect of the DIPJ and the patient is unable to flex the joint.

A similar mechanism of injury can result in a tear of the flexor tendon pulleys that bind the tendon to the proximal phalanx. Active flexion is intact but there is pain with tenderness over the mid-proximal phalanx area. The flexor tendon may 'bowstring' on resisted flexion.

Management
Discuss FDP rupture with specialty teams, as local practice may vary with regard to further imaging (magnetic resonance imaging, MRI) and early surgical intervention. Flexor pulley injuries are usually treated conservatively with reduction in activity and taping.

Proximal interphalangeal joint (PIPJ) injuries
Introduction
PIPJ injuries are common and frequently frustrating for both the patient and the attending clinician. The main source of frustration is the totally unpredictable nature of their clinical course which seems unrelated to the severity of the original injury.

The PIPJ is stabilized by the extensor and flexor tendons, radial and ulnar collateral ligaments, the joint capsule and a very strong ligament on the volar aspect of the joint: the volar plate. Injuries disrupt one or more of these elements and are frequently associated with a small avulsion fracture from the volar aspect of the base of the middle phalanx.

Presentation can range from minor bruising or swelling to complete dislocation. The mechanism is most frequently hyperextension or axial loading. There is usually pain, bruising, deformity, swelling and bony injury as above. There may also be instability, haemarthrosis and, rarely, an acute extensor tendon rupture resulting in a traumatic boutonniere deformity.

Management
It is often difficult to adequately assess these injuries at initial presentation because the pain is often intense and disproportionate to

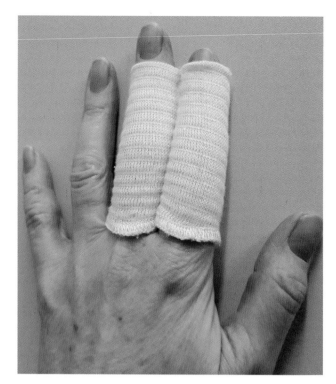

Figure 8.3 Bedford splint.

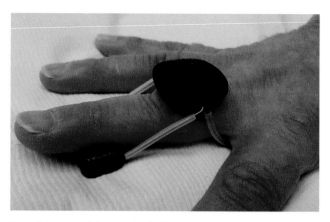

Figure 8.4 Armchair (boutonniere) splint.

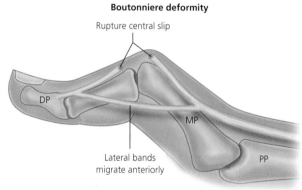

Boutonniere deformity

Rupture central slip

DP

MP

PP

Lateral bands
migrate anteriorly

1. Central slip rupture
2. Over 7-10 days lateral bands migrate anteriorly
3. PIPJ "Buttonholes" through gap

Figure 8.5 Boutonniere deformity.

the apparent injury. Emergency department management consists of analgesia (including high-arm sling), plain radiography and a Bedford splint or equivalent for 3–4 days (Figure 8.3). All patients should be advised to commence mobilization exercises as soon as possible. More specific interventions are outlined here.

Reduction of a dislocated or subluxed PIPJ

If clinically or radiographically confirmed, these injuries should be manipulated as a matter of urgency. They are usually relatively easy to reduce by axial traction using Entonox or digital nerve block.

Specialty review

If an acute boutonniere deformity or large fracture fragment is identified, it is appropriate to discuss with inpatient teams although it is highly unlikely that any of these injuries would require acute operative intervention.

Follow-up

All these injuries should be reviewed within 2–3 weeks because of the difficulties in assessing them at initial presentation and their unpredictable recovery period and final functional outcome. The mainstay of ongoing treatment is physiotherapy including mobilization, banding to reduce swelling, dynamic splinting with 'armchair' or boutonniere splints (Figure 8.4) and referral to a hand specialist in cases not responding to conservative management.

Boutonniere injury

Acute traumatic rupture of the middle slip of the extensor tendon over the PIPJ is hard to diagnose. The history is of a blow to the dorsum of the PIPJ when the finger is flexed, for example pushing hard on a spanner that slips, causing the knuckle to hit the edge of an engine. This causes blunt rupture of the central slip. However, as the lateral bands are still intact over the dorsum of the joint, the patient can still extend the PIPJ. Over the next 1–2 weeks, with repeated normal finger flexion, the lateral bands migrate around to the sides of the joint and the head of the PP 'buttonholes' through the tendon, hence the name 'boutonniere' deformity (Figure 8.5).

Diagnosis

The clinical diagnosis of a central slip injury is difficult. In a patient with the mechanism of injury described above and pain swelling and tenderness over the dorsum of the PIPJ, the finger should be splinted in extension and referred for review or for an ultrasound scan.

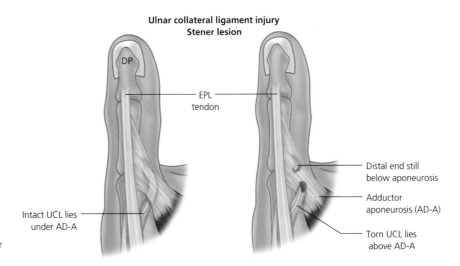

Ulnar collateral ligament injury
Stener lesion

DP

EPL
tendon

Distal end still
below aponeurosis

Adductor
aponeurosis (AD-A)

Intact UCL lies
under AD-A

Torn UCL lies
above AD-A

Figure 8.6 UCL injury: Stener lesion. ADA, adductor aponeurosis.

Treatment

If a central slip rupture is confirmed then the patient is treated initially in an extension splint and then in an armchair splint (Figure 8.4) that allows some flexion but always returns the finger to an extended position. Such injuries are usually followed up in a hand clinic.

Ulnar collateral ligament (UCL) injuries of the thumb

Introduction

Stability of the metacarpo-phalangeal joint (MCPJ) of the thumb is maintained by strong adductor and opponens muscles and the UCL of the MCPJ. The injuries may be due to chronic abduction stress (gamekeeper's thumb) or forced abduction while holding an object (skier's thumb). The ligament may be sprained, partially torn or ruptured.

Patients present with an acutely painful, swollen thumb MCPJ, which may be unstable when the UCL is stressed. However, it is often too painful to fully assess the extent of any instability at initial presentation. Wrist and thumb movements are often maintained.

When the ligament tears completely, the torn ends may become separated by the aponeurosis of adductor policis (Stener lesion), which has implications for outcome and management (Figure 8.6).

Management

As clinical examination is unreliable in predicting the severity of injury at initial presentation, management in the emergency department is directed towards pain relief and protecting the joint from further damage. Plain radiography should be performed to identify any associated bony injury. An attempt should be made to assess the stability of the MCPJ by stressing the UCL in both extension and 30° of flexion. Local anaesthetic may help.

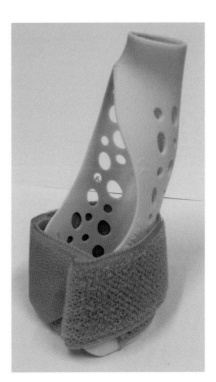

Figure 8.7 Plastic thumb spica for UCL injury.

Immobilization

In the vast majority of cases the thumb MCPJ should be immobilized using a removable thermoplastic thumb spica (Figure 8.7). If these are not available place the thumb in a shortened scaphoid plaster. Elastoplast thumb spicas are ineffective.

Further imaging on initial presentation

For any patient who clearly has a completely ruptured UCL on initial presentation, or if the patient's occupation or high-level performance depends on optimal functioning of this joint, an urgent MRI or ultrasound should be arranged.

Specialty review

Any patient who is considered for urgent MRI or ultrasound, or in whom a Stener lesion is suspected, should be discussed with a specialist team according to local protocols. These patients may benefit from surgical repair of the ligament within a week of sustaining the injury.

Follow-up

All these injuries should be reviewed within 5–7 days because of the difficulties in assessing them at initial presentation. At this time it is easier to assess instability, decide whether the splint is still performing a useful function and evaluate the need for any physiotherapy or surgical intervention.

Further reading

Kacprowicz RF, Ho SW. Ulnar collateral ligament injury. http://emedicine .medscape.com/article/97451 (accessed 14 December 2015).

Rosh AJ, Schraga E. Extensor tendon repair. http://emedicine.medscape.com/ article/109111 (accessed 14 December 2015).

Wardrope J, English B. *Musculo-skeletal problems in emergency medicine.* Oxford University Press, Oxford, 1998.

CHAPTER 9

Common Soft Tissue Disorders of the Hip

Alison Smeatham

Royal Devon & Exeter Hospital, Exeter, UK

With contributions from Rahul Anaspure, Royal Devon & Exeter Hospital, Exeter, UK

OVERVIEW

- This chapter covers diagnosis and treatment of common soft tissue injuries around the hip.
- The descriptions will enable the practitioner to identify chronic soft tissue injuries around the hip and consider underlying causative factors.
- The planning of treatment for soft tissue injuries around the hip is described.
- Alternative differential diagnoses of hip pain are outlined.

Soft tissue disorders around the hip occur as isolated lesions, particularly in the athletic population. However, in any case of ongoing hip or thigh pain, associated spinal, pelvic and hip joint pathology should be considered. Poor spinal flexibility and stability, faulty lower limb biomechanics and muscle imbalance commonly contribute to ongoing symptoms and should be considered throughout assessment and treatment. See Box 9.1.

Tendinopathies and muscle lesions

As in other commonly affected sites of the musculoskeletal system, contractile lesions around the hip can occur suddenly, associated with trauma or as recurrent or chronic lesions.

General principles of treatment
Acute muscle and tendon injury

Prompt treatment of acute lesions is based on the 'POLICE' regime (Bleakley *et al.* 2012) of **p**rotection, **o**ptimum **l**oading, **i**ce, **c**ompression and **e**levation supplemented by simple analgesia. Protection in the first 48 hours post-injury includes avoidance of aggravating activities, and in severe cases may warrant use of crutches. Compression of the structures around the hip can be achieved by use of strapping, compressive hosiery or shorts.

Box 9.1 **Differential diagnosis of disorders around the hip**

Common causes
Acute muscle strains: adductors, hamstrings
Occult fracture
Chronic tendinopthies: adductors, hamstrings, glutei, iliopsoas
Bursitis: trochanteric, psoas
Referred pain from the lumbar spine and sacroiliac joints
Osteoarthritis of the hip
Inguinal hernia

Less common causes
Femoroacetabular impingement
Chondral lesions
Femoral or sports hernia,
Osteitis pubis
Perthes disease
Slipped upper femoral epiphysis
Irritable hip
Hip dysplasia

Rare but important causes
Stress fracture of the pelvis or femur
Avascular necrosis of the femoral head
Referred pain from the viscera
Apophysitis or avulsion fracture
Secondary or primary tumour
Psoas abcess
Inflammatory arthritis

Optimum loading in the very early stages after injury reduces the load through injured structures. Loading is progressed as healing occurs by increasing range of movement, force, stretch, velocity and function with the aim of returning the patient and injured structure to full pain-free activity.

Graded progressive rehabilitation starts immediately with pain-free active movement of the hip, knee and spinal joints, static contraction of the major unaffected muscle groups, and a programme to maintain fitness and gait re-education. After approximately 48 hours, the range of active hip movement can increase, contraction of the affected contractile unit can commence, and proprioceptive exercises added, all of which should be performed within pain-free limits. Over the ensuing days and

ABC of Common Soft Tissue Disorders, First Edition.
Edited by Francis Morris, Jim Wardrope and Paul Hattam.
© 2016 John Wiley & Sons, Ltd. Published 2016 by John Wiley & Sons, Ltd.

weeks rehabilitation is progressed to include open and closed-chain exercise, eccentric and concentric strengthening, change in pace, direction, acceleration, deceleration and stretches of the injured structure.

Chronic and recurrent tendinopathy

Chronic and recurrent tendinopathy around the hip is associated with degenerative change within the connective tissue of the tendon. This may be as a result of an ineffectively managed acute injury or secondary to biomechanical overload. Although research specific to the hip is lacking, the principles of treatment can be assumed from other areas commonly affected by tendinopathy; that is, initial activity modulation, gradual loading and fitness training. Adjunctative treatments such as corticosteroid injection, non-steroidal anti-inflammatory drugs (NSAIDs) and shockwave therapy (lithotripsy) can be used to facilitate rehabilitation. Modalities such as autologous blood or platelet-rich plasma injection are untested around the hip.

Adductor tendinopathy

History

Acute adductor lesions commonly occur in footballers where a rapid change of direction is accompanied by the sudden onset of groin pain. If continued activity is possible, the pain is aggravated by acceleration/deceleration, lateral cutting or running over rough ground.

Recurrent or chronic adductor-related groin pain can be challenging to diagnose and manage. The differential diagnosis in ongoing conditions includes femoroacetabular impingement, hip joint osteoarthritis, hernia, osteitis pubis, stress fracture, psoas tendinopathy and bursitis, or referred pain from the spine, sacroiliac joint or viscera.

Examination

The adductor longus is most commonly affected at its origin at the body of the pubis or within the musculotendinous junction. The affected site is tender to palpation.

Full hip joint movement should be possible once acute pain has subsided. Resisted contraction and stretching of the hip adductors will be painful. Recurrent and chronic conditions require a more extensive examination of the spine, pelvis, sacroiliac joint and symphysis pubis.

Investigations

Investigation is not routinely required in simple acute lesions unless they fail to respond to treatment. Ultrasound scan will outline tendon lesions and also aid differential diagnosis in distinguishing hernias. Bone scintigraphy will isolate active bone turnover in osteitis pubis which can accompany adductor tendon lesions. In chronic conditions, a range of investigations including magnetic resonance imaging (MRI) may be needed to exclude other possible causes of pain.

Box 9.2 **Rehabilitation programme for adductor tendinopathy**

Module I (first 2 weeks)
1 Static adduction against soccer ball placed between feet when lying supine; each adduction 30 s, 10 repetitions.
2 Static adduction against soccer ball placed between knees when lying supine; each adduction 30s, 10 repetitions.
3 Abdominal sit-ups in both straightforward direction and oblique direction; five series of 10 repetitions.
4 Combined abdominal sit-up and hip flexion, starting from supine position and with soccer ball placed between knees (folding knife exercise); five series of 10 repetitions.
5 Balance training on wobble board for 5 minutes.
6 One-foot exercises on sliding board, with parallel feet as well as with 90° angle between feet; five sets of 1 minute's continuous work with each leg, and in both positions.

Module II (from third week; module II is done twice at each training session)
1 Leg abduction and adduction exercises lying on side; five series of 10 repetitions of each exercise.
2 Low-back extension exercises prone over end of couch; five series of 10 repetitions.
3 One-leg weight-pulling abduction/adduction standing; five series of 10 repetitions for each leg.
4 Abdominal sit-ups in both straightforward direction and oblique direction; five series of 10 repetitions.
5 One-leg coordination exercise flexing and extending knee and swinging arms in same rhythm (cross country skiing on one leg); five series of 10 repetitions for each leg.
6 Training in sidewards motion on a 'fitter' (rocking base curved on top and bottom; user stands on platform that rolls laterally on tracks on top of rocking base) for 5 min.
7 Balance training on wobble board for 5 minutes.
8 Skating movements on sliding board; five times 1 minute's continuous work.

From Holmich et al. (1999).

Treatment

The principles of treatment are outlined earlier in the chapter. An 8–12-week rehabilitation programme aimed at improving the muscular stability of the pelvis, hips and adductor muscles has been shown to improve outcomes in athletes with chronic adductor pain (Box 9.2).

Referral for further investigation should be considered in complex cases that fail to respond to treatment or where there is diagnostic uncertainty.

Hip flexor tendinopathy

History

The attachments of the psoas to the lumbar spine and lesser trochanter mean that it can be linked with both back and groin pain, however the patient usually notices deep anterior hip pain on active hip flexion such as kicking a football or climbing stairs.

Following total hip arthroplasty, direct impingement of the tendon from the prostheses can cause external pressure on the tendon.

Overuse, weakness or shortening of the psoas can cause pain. The psoas tendon sheath may communicate with the hip joint as can the psoas bursa, and so mixed lesions affecting all these structures may occur.

A sudden onset is unusual and lumbar discitis or psoas abscess should be considered if the presentation is acute and unexplained particularly if accompanied by systemic illness or fever. Psoas tendon problems are unusual in children and adolescents and other causes of pain should be excluded; for example apophysitis, irritable hip, Perthes disease, slipped capital femoral epiphysis, avulsion and stress fractures.

Examination

Tenderness can be palpated at the tendon insertion to the lesser trochanter.

Passive hip extension may be limited and painful. Tightness of the psoas, and the other structures anterior to the hip can be further assessed with Thomas test (Figure 9.1).

Resisted hip flexion tested with hip joint at 90° flexion reproduces the patient's familiar groin pain. As the leg is returned to the couch, the psoas tendon may be felt to 'clunk' over the femoral head.

Investigations

MRI of the lumbar spine and pelvis allows assessment of the psoas and also other possible causes of pain in the spine and abdomen.

Treatment

Principles of treatment for acute and chronic hip tendons are outlined above.

In psoas tendinopathy particular attention is focused on addressing loss of muscular stability around the pelvis and spine. The addition of manipulative therapy to the lumbar spine, soft tissue mobilization, anterior hip stretches and a graduated strengthening programme are added as indicated. In refractory cases, image-guided injection to the psoas can be helpful diagnostically and therapeutically.

Hamstring tendinopathy

History

Contractile lesions of the hamstrings are amongst the most commonly encountered soft tissue lesions in the lower limb. They occur in many sports, particularly hurdles, sprinting, hockey and football, where they comprise 12% of all injuries. Recurrent or chronic hamstring lesions can involve the muscle belly or the teno-osseous origin at the ischial tuberosity.

The patient often makes the correct diagnosis themselves, particularly when the onset is sudden. Sharp onset of posterior thigh pain usually occurs during the terminal swing phase when sprinting. The patient may be unable to continue their activity and extensive bruising/haematoma may be observed within 24 hours.

Although diagnosis is usually straightforward, referred pain from the lumbar spine and sacroiliac joint should be considered in chronic conditions. Pain felt at the ischial origin may accompany ischial bursitis which can co-exist with lesions at the hamstring origin. In adolescents, apophysitis or avulsion of the ischial tuberosity can mimic an acute hamstring origin lesion.

Vascular claudication can cause exercise-related posterior thigh pain.

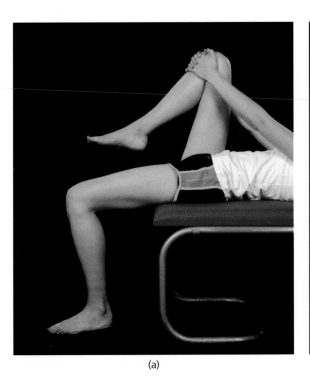 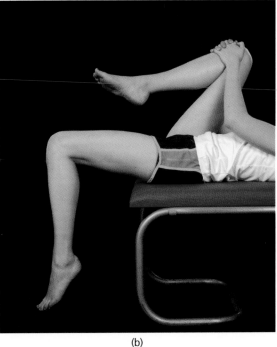

(a)   (b)

Figure 9.1 Thomas test.

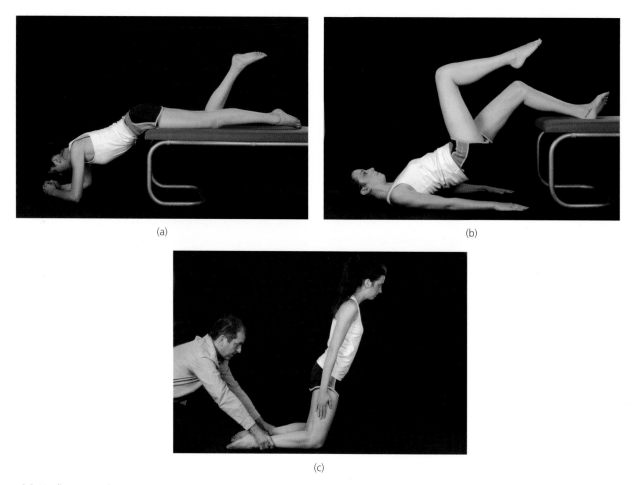

(a)

(b)

(c)

Figure 9.2 Nordic eccentric hamstring exercise.

Examination

In acute lesions of the muscle belly, extensive bruising can be observed over the posterior thigh. The patient will be reluctant to stretch the hamstrings and so will avoid full knee extension combined with hip flexion when walking.

Tenderness is palpable at the site of the lesion and as swelling dissipates a palpable gap at the site of the muscle tear may be apparent.

In acute and chronic cases, straight leg raise is limited and painful. Resisted contraction of the hamstrings during hip extension and knee flexion produces pain, and there is tenderness at the site of the lesion.

Investigations

Investigations are rarely required but ultrasound scanning can confirm the site and extent of the lesion with the added benefit of enabling a guided diagnostic or therapeutic injection. MRI will outline the contractile lesion and provide additional information to aid differential diagnosis.

Treatment

Principles of treatment for acute and chronic hip tendons are outlined above. In acute lesions, the POLICE regime, gentle transverse friction massage, strapping and a graduated exercise programme should be implemented quickly to ensure rapid, complete recovery and prevention of chronicity.

At a later stage of healing, or in chronic conditions, inclusion of strengthening exercises for the gluteal and adductor magnus muscles and eccentric muscle exercises are recommended, for example Nordic training (Figure 9.2). Return to competitive sport follows once full hip and knee movement, concentric and eccentric strength and the ability to perform all components of the chosen sport in training are achieved.

Clinical tip

Injuries to the origin of the hamstring muscles usually occur in athletes and can result in an *avulsion fracture* of the ischium or a pure avulsion of the hamstring tendons themselves, depending on the patient's age. These are rare injuries and are often initially misdiagnosed as a simple hamstring 'pull', which can lead to persistent symptoms. X-ray and/or MRI will elucidate.

Trochanteric tendinopathy and bursitis
History

This common cause of lateral hip pain may occur in the younger active population as a result of overuse and pain may be accompanied by a 'snapping' sensation of the iliotibial band. However, it is more common in a sedentary older population. There is increasing evidence that trochanteric bursitis is rare in the absence of underlying gluteal tendinopathy and the term greater trochanteric pain syndrome (GTPS) is increasingly used to signify a combination of tendinopathy, bursitis and referred pain from the spine and sacroiliac joint.

Typically, a gradual onset of lateral hip pain is noted after unaccustomed activity. This is exacerbated by climbing stairs or slopes and pain can cause sleep disturbance when the patient lies on the affected hip.

Examination

A Trendelenberg gait or positive Trendlenberg test may be observed: as the patient stands on their affected leg, the pelvis on the contralateral side dips as gluteal strength is insufficient to maintain the body weight over the limb (Figure 9.3).

Tenderness is felt on palpation of the lateral or posterior aspects of the greater trochanter. Passive hip movement may lack the last few degrees of straight leg raise, external rotation, flexion and adduction as the gluteal structures are stretched or compressed. Resisted hip abduction is painful and often weak.

Investigations

Ultrasound examination will identify a tendon tear and fluid within the trochanteric bursae and allow a simultaneous image-guided injection. MRI will provide similar information.

Treatment

Principles of treatment for chronic hip tendons are outlined above. A graduated programme is initiated to strengthen the gluteal muscles in combination with exercises to improve core stability of the pelvis and spine. In the short term, a steroid/local anaesthetic injection to the greater trochanter can provide good, if short-term, pain relief. Shockwave therapy may be considered in resistant cases in some centres. Treatment of associated spinal and biomechanical factors should also be considered.

Piriformis impingement

The piriformis is a deep external rotator of the hip, attaching to the sacrum and passing to the greater trochanter. As it does so, it passes superficially to the sciatic nerve but in approximately 10% of the population the nerve passes through the muscle where it can become impinged, resulting in local buttock pain and referred pain with paraesthesia in the distribution of the sciatic nerve. Similar symptoms can occur after traumatic soft tissue injuries to the buttock.

Piriformis syndrome is a more commonly used term for non-specific buttock pain with trigger points in the pelvic and buttock region. Every effort should be made to diagnose the underlying cause of pain. This may be referred from the spine and sacroiliac joint or secondary to weakness, tightness or overuse of the deep hip external rotators which are often associated with poor spinal and pelvic stability and reduced activity of the stronger gluteal muscles.

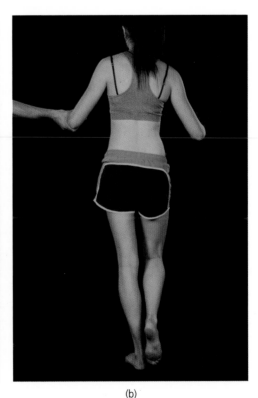

(a) (b)

Figure 9.3 Trendelenberg test.

History and examination

Piriformis impingement may be caused by trauma to the buttock, causing pain that is sometimes accompanied by paraesthesia in the calf and foot. This occurs when sitting or when the piriformis is stretched in hip flexion and adduction, for example when sitting with the leg crossed. If symptoms are reproduced on palpation of the sciatic nerve at the greater sciatic notch, nerve impingement at the site of piriformis is suspected.

In Piriformis syndrome, the history is often inconclusive and diffuse buttock pain is felt but paraesthesia is not reported. On palpation, tender trigger spots are felt in the gluteal muscles and deeper external rotators between the lateral edge of the sacrum and greater trochanter.

Passive hip flexion, adduction and internal rotation stretch the piriformis and reproduce the patient's pain. Resisted external rotation of the hip activates all the external rotators and may reproduce pain.

Investigations

Asymmetry of the piriformis muscle bulk on MRI or computed tomography (CT) scan may suggest impingement. An electromyogram (EMG) can assist if a diagnosis of sciatic nerve impingement is being considered and the site of impingement is uncertain.

Treatment

In cases of piriformis impingement, soft tissue mobilization and piriformis and gluteal stretches may be sufficient to alleviate symptoms. Further investigation and surgical exploration may be considered in refractory cases. In cases of piriformis syndrome, treatment is directed to the underlying cause, for example lumbar spine referral, muscle weakness or tightness.

Other hip disorders

Meralgia paraesthetica

History

Compression of the lateral femoral cutaneous nerve of the thigh as it passes under the lateral aspect of the inguinal ligament can cause well-defined sensory disturbance over the anterior aspect of

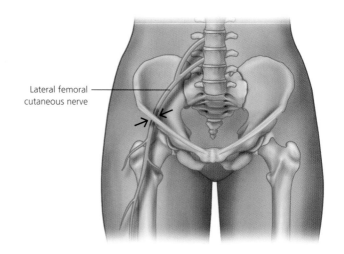

Lateral femoral cutaneous nerve

Figure 9.4 Distribution of numbness in the thigh.

the thigh. This is known as meralgia paraesthetica. Trauma and direct pressure caused by obesity or tight-fitting clothing may be contributory factors.

Examination

The patient presents with a well-defined area of numbness over the anterolateral aspect of the thigh and no motor deficit. Palpation over the lateral femoral cutaneous nerve as it passes slightly medial to the anterior superior iliac spine may reproduce the symptoms. See Figure 9.4.

Investigations

Investigations may not be required provided the diagnosis is straightforward. However, an ultrasound scan is helpful in identifying anatomical variations of the inguinal ligament and nerve.

Treatment

The symptoms can resolve over time once the causative agents are removed. Image-guided injection of steroid and local anaesthetic adjacent to the nerve as it exits from under the inguinal ligament is usually curative.

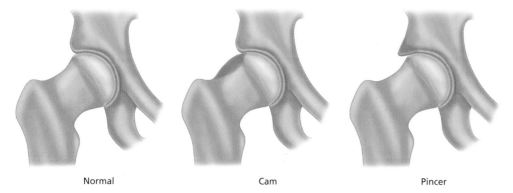

Normal   Cam   Pincer

Figure 9.5 Cam and pincer deformities.

Acetabular labrum lesions/femoroacetabular impingement

History

There is increasing awareness that acetabular labral lesions can cause hip joint pain in adults under the age of 50. Femoro-acetabular impingement can be caused by morphological changes of the femoral head–neck junction (Cam impingement) or pathology of the labrum (Pincer impingement). (see Figure 9.5).

The patient's main complaint is of groin and/or lateral hip pain particularly on hip flexion activities such as sitting, squatting. Onset may be linked with trauma but is just as often of gradual onset.

Examination

On examination, the pain is most consistently reproduced with combined hip flexion, adduction and internal rotation (FAIR test) (Figure 9.6).

Investigations

X-ray may reveal abnormalities, often subtle, of the femoral head–neck junction. Magnetic resonance arthrogram provides further information on the bony morphology and acetabular labrum and also excludes other pathologies.

Treatment

Initial treatment is conservative. Physiotherapy is aimed at addressing movement abnormalities and muscle imbalance. If ineffective, image-guided steroid and local anaesthetic injection can be helpful diagnostically and therapeutically. Resistant cases are increasingly treated by arthroscopic hip surgery.

Osteoarthritis of the hip

History

Although not a soft tissue disorder, osteoarthritis of the hip should be considered in the differential diagnosis of pain around the hip. Middle-aged and older individuals present with gradually worsening groin, lateral or buttock pain, which can refer to anterior aspect of thigh, knee and shin.

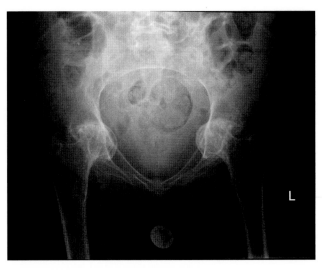

Figure 9.7 X-ray of osteoarthritis of the hip.

Examination

On examination, a painful limp may be apparent and is most noticeable on the first few steps after rising from sitting. The range of hip movement is limited, particularly internal rotation, flexion and abduction.

Investigations

X-ray of the pelvis confirms the diagnosis (Figure 9.7).

Treatment

Treatment guidelines have been published by the National Institute for Health and Care Excellence (2008). In the initial stages pain relief, weight loss and exercise are recommended. Total hip arthroplasty is considered when pain relief is not obtained with conservative treatment.

Further reading

Bleakley CM, Glasgow P, MacAuley DC. PRICE need updating, should we call the POLICE? *Br J Sports Med* 2012;**46**:220–221.

Brukner P, Khan K. *Clinical sports medicine*, 4th edn. McGraw-Hill Medical, Australia, 2012.

Hattam P, Smeatham A. *Special tests in musculoskeletal examination: an evidence-based guide for clinicians*. Churchill Livingstone, London, 2010.

Holmich P, Uhrskou P, Ulnits L *et al.* Effectiveness of active physical training for long standing adductor related groin pain in athletes: a randomised trial. *Lancet* 1999;**353**:439–443.

National Institute for Health and Care Excellence (NICE). *The care and management of osteoarthritis in adults CG59*. NICE, London, 2008.

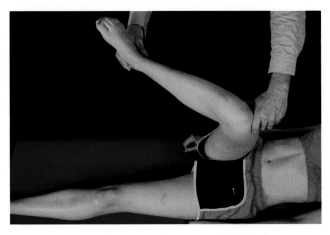

Figure 9.6 The 'FAIR' (flexion, internal rotation and adduction) test.

CHAPTER 10

Soft Tissue Knee Injuries

Paul M. Sutton

Sheffield Orthopaedics Ltd, Sheffield, UK

OVERVIEW

- This chapter outlines history taking and examination in knee injury.
- It gives advice on the triage of acute knee injury.
- Outlines are given of the management of cruciate ligament injury, collateral ligament injury and patellar dislocation.

Box 10.1 **Key points in examination of acute knee injury**

Can the patient walk?

Is there deformity?

Is there specific bony tenderness?

Is there an effusion?

Can the patient perform a straight leg raise?

Are there signs of ligamentous instability?

Are distal pulses, sensation and power intact?

Introduction

Soft tissue knee injuries are common as the knee is particularly susceptible to injury because of its peripheral position, subcutaneous location and a relative lack of bony constraint. There is evidence that significant soft tissue knee injuries may be neglected and misdiagnosed. There is also evidence that maltreatment of a significant soft tissue injury may lead to further preventable knee damage. This chapter focuses on the common soft tissue knee injuries.

The approach to knee injury and knee injury triage

History

The mechanism of injury can often indicate the likely pathology. Sports injuries are a particularly common cause of major soft tissue injury. Immediate swelling indicates a haemarthrosis. True locking and true giving way should be distinguished from pseudo-locking and functional giving way. True locking means the patient is unable to fully extend, but a more typical presentation is of intermittent episodes of locking associated with a manouevre to 'unlock' the joint, often with a clunking sound or sensation. Pseudo-locking is a sudden pain with difficulty flexing and extending the knee; these symptoms gradually ease without the abrupt mechanical release noted with true locking. Pseudo-locking is caused by pain and is commonly described in patients with osteoarthritis. True giving way typically occurs with an abrupt change of direction such as during pivoting sports or walking over uneven terrain. This is often due to a ligament injury. Functional giving way is associated

with quadriceps weakness or pain where the patient feels the knee 'gives'. It may occur with straight-line activities and usually does not cause a fall.

Previous problems or injuries are important to note.

Examination

Follow the look, feel, move system. Examine the hip as referred pain is a common cause of error in patients presenting with knee pain. Specific tests for each injury are discussed below but the questions in Box 10.1 need to be addressed.

Does the patient need an x-ray?

In most significant knee injuries an x-ray is required. However, the Ottawa knee rules indicate that if the patient is younger than 55 years, can weight bear at the time of injury and take four steps in the emergency department, can flex to 90° and has no tenderness over the fibular head or patella then x-ray can be deferred but the patient advised to return if symptoms get worse.

Triage of knee injury

Figure 10.1 outlines a scheme for the triage of knee injuries. This can only be a rough guide: each patient should be treated according to the findings on history, examination and x-rays.

Cruciate ligament injuries

The anterior cruciate ligament (ACL) lies in the centre of the knee within the femoral notch. It originates from the tibial plateau between the tibial spines, runs obliquely and inserts on the medial

ABC of Common Soft Tissue Disorders, First Edition.
Edited by Francis Morris, Jim Wardrope and Paul Hattam.

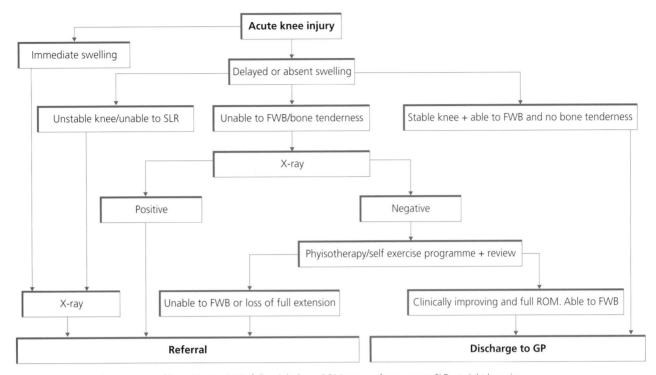

Figure 10.1 A scheme for the triage of knee injuries. FWB, full weight bear; ROM, range of movement; SLR, straight leg raise.

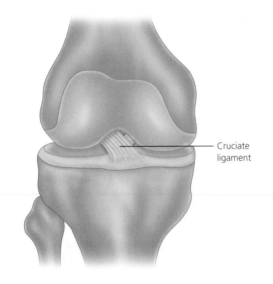

Figure 10.2 Cruciate ligaments.

aspect of the lateral femoral condyle. The posterior cruciate ligament (PCL) also runs within the femoral notch from the central posterior border of the proximal tibia upwards to the anterolateral aspect of the medial femoral condyle. The ACL crosses anteriorly to the PCL, and together they form a cross structure (Figure 10.2).

These ligaments act in synergy, directing knee movement. Together they contribute significantly to the knee's stability. The PCL is thicker than the ACL. It acts to prevent posterior movement of the tibia relative to the femur. The ACL prevents anterior

movement of tibia relative to the femur but more importantly contributes to the rotational stability of the knee.

ACL injuries
History
Injury to the ACL is common and often misdiagnosed. The injury typically occurs during sports that involve landing from a jump or sudden directional change. The classic ACL injury mechanism is a valgus and external rotation force that the patient describes as a twisting injury.

Other features in the history may be a twisting mechanism over a planted foot, a fall to the ground, the sensation of a pop or crack from the knee, the knee moving in an abnormal manner, sudden and significant knee pain, difficulty weight bearing and inability to continue playing their sport.

The ACL is a vascular structure and bleeds following injury, leading to a haemarthrosis, which the patient will note as rapid knee swelling. This may be contrasted with other soft tissue injuries that do not cause acute bleeding but may be associated with gradual swelling due to inflammation and a reactive synovitis.

Examination
The anterior draw test is described to detect ACL rupture; however, there is large false negative rate associated with this test. Evidence suggests that the sensitivity of the anterior draw test may be as low as 50%. A more accurate test of ACL function is the Lachman test (Figure 10.3). This is similar to the anterior draw test except that the anterior force is applied with the knee at approximately 10–20° of flexion rather than 90°. Note the degree of anterior movement

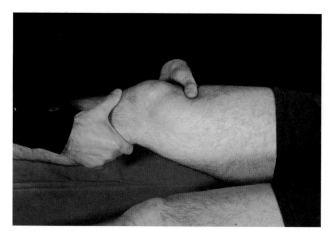

Figure 10.3 The Lachman test. Note the degree of flexion and the hand position, allowing an anterior force on the proximal tibia.

and the presence or absence of an 'end point'. Compare the degree of movement between the injured and un-injured knee. After acute ACL rupture clinical assessment may be difficult due to pain and guarding. If an ACL injury is suspected bring the patient back for early review and consider magnetic resonance imaging (MRI), a sensitive investigation for acute ACL rupture.

Treatment

The initial management of an ACL injury is aimed at reducing swelling and restoring a full range of movement and muscle function as quickly as possible to prevent secondary muscle wasting. Advise simple compression, analgesia and regular icing. Crutches may be required for pain relief. This management should be followed by early referral for physiotherapy and a specialist opinion. Immediate surgical intervention is rarely necessary and some patients with a rupture of the ACL will require no surgical treatment. Patients who have ongoing symptoms of instability despite

appropriate rehabilitation may require surgical treatment. This typically involves reconstructing the ruptured ligament with a biological graft and usually allows a successful return to pre-injury function.

PCL injuries

This ligament is injured far less frequently than the ACL. When it occurs, it is usually due to a posterior blow to the proximal tibia with the knee flexed, for example a dashboard impact in a road traffic accident. The PCL is intra-articular but extra-synovial so although vascular rupture may not be associated with a haemarthrosis it can lead to visible bruising in the calf. Patients often describe less severe initial symptoms following PCL rupture compared to ACL injury. After sports-related PCL injury patients are usually unable to continue playing and weight bearing may be difficult. The injury can usually be confirmed by clinical examination. The easiest method of detecting a PCL injury is to flex both knees to 90° and view the knees from the side, specifically examining the proximal tibia and tibial tuberosity (Figure 10.4). Following a PCL injury the proximal tibia will sag posteriorly compared with the normal knee. This may be confirmed by applying a posterior force, known as the posterior draw test.

For patients with an isolated PCL injury the mainstay of treatment is non-operative. The initial management is aimed at improving swelling and restoring movement followed by a formal quadriceps muscle-strengthening programme. The PCL has some potential to heal and this may be helped with the continuous use of a protective brace for up to 3 months. The role of surgical management of an isolated PCL rupture is controversial as there is mixed evidence that surgery results in better outcomes than non-operative treatment.

When assessing a cruciate injury exclude associated ligament damage as both ACL and PCL rupture may occur in combination with other injuries. Any injured knee with signs suggestive of a multiple ligament injury should be immobilized and an urgent

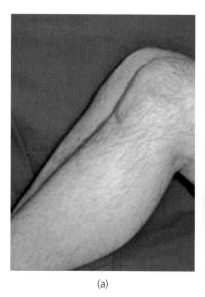
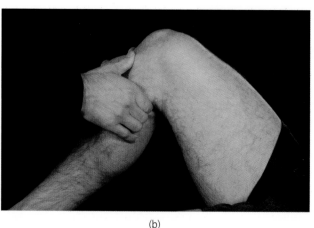

(a)   (b)

Figure 10.4 Detecting a PCL injury. Note the posterior sag of the proximal tibia (a) and the posterior force applied for the posterior draw test (b).

specialist opinion sought. Multiple ligament injury can lead to a complete tibiofemoral dislocation, which is a rare injury that may be missed as it is often associated with spontaneous relocation. Most patients who sustain this injury have clinical evidence of gross instability and there is a high risk of associated popliteal artery injury, a limb threatening complication.

Medial collateral ligament (MCL)

The MCL traverses the medial aspect of the knee from the bony prominence of the medial femoral epicondyle to the anteromedial surface of the proximal tibia. The ligament resists an abnormal separation of the medial tibiofemoral compartment. It is a complex structure comprising different components that function at different degrees of flexion.

History

An accurate history of the injury mechanism is the key to diagnosing MCL injury. The MCL is the most commonly injured knee ligament, and injury occurs as a consequence of a valgus force. This may arise due to a laterally directed force applied to the distal limb or foot, for example in a skiing injury. It may also occur due to a medially directed force applied to the outside of the knee in a weight-bearing leg, for example an impact while playing contact sport.

Examination

The MCL is an extra-articular structure so a significant joint effusion is unusual and if noted is likely to indicate an associated injury such as rupture of the ACL. Localized medial swelling may be noted. The ligament can be injured at any point along its length but will be maximally painful and tender at the site of injury. Assess the integrity of the MCL by applying a valgus stress with the knee slightly flexed (Figure 10.5). On applying load to an injured MCL the patient will experience pain, which helps confirm the diagnosis. Compare the laxity with the un-injured knee. With a grade 1 injury there is no abnormal laxity of the MCL: this may be considered a minor sprain-type injury. A grade 2 injury is determined by mild to moderate laxity of the MCL but there is a point at which the ligament resists further abnormal motion, referred to as an end point. This injury may be considered a partial rupture of the MCL. Grade 3 injuries are determined by significant laxity of the MCL and no end point. This injury is a complete rupture of the MCL and is frequently associated with other ligament damage, most commonly the ACL.

Treatment

The initial management of a MCL injury is aimed at reducing inflammation and restoring movement. This may be achieved with advice, ice treatment and early physiotherapy. All MCL injuries have the potential to heal spontaneously, allowing a return to excellent function. However, grade 3 injuries require protection to facilitate this healing. This is achieved by placing the injured knee in a hinged brace (Figure 10.6). Full weight bearing is allowed

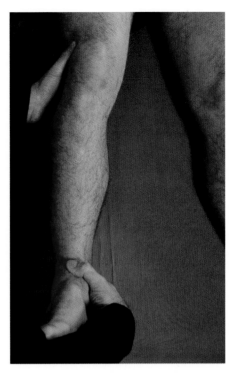

Figure 10.5 Assessing the integrity of the MCL. Note the hand position controlling the knee and permitting the application of a valgus force.

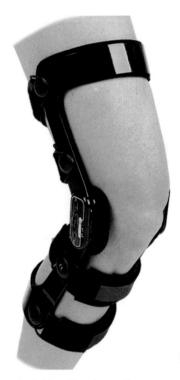

Figure 10.6 A simple hinged knee brace allows movement but protects the MCL.

but the amount of permitted knee movement is controversial. The author permits a full range of motion.

Isolated MCL injuries rarely require surgery. However, MCL injuries associated with other ligament damage are more likely to require surgical intervention.

Lateral collateral ligament (LCL)

The LCL runs down the lateral aspect of the knee from the bony prominence of the lateral femoral epicondyle to the head of the fibula. It is a small structure of just a few millimetres diameter. Its primary function is to prevent abnormal opening of the lateral tibiofemoral compartment. LCL injury is uncommon but when injured is frequently injured in association with other ligaments. Complete rupture of the LCL is also associated with a high risk of peroneal nerve injury that will manifest clinically as a footdrop.

History

The diagnosis of a LCL injury can usually be established by the injury mechanism, combined with lateral pain and possible symptoms of instability. It is injured when an excessive varus force is applied to the leg.

Examination

The LCL is extra-articular so swelling associated with this injury is typically localized to the lateral side of the knee rather than an effusion. The injured ligament will be tender. With a varus stress there will be lateral-sided pain and possible laxity. Assessment of ligament laxity is best performed at 20–30° of knee flexion and the degree of laxity is determined by the severity of the injury.

Treatment

Treatment of LCL laxity after acute injury should consist of protecting the knee joint with a splint and prompt referral for a specialist opinion. In contrast to the MCL the LCL has little potential to heal spontaneously and for significant LCL injuries early surgical exploration is usually recommended. Early surgery allows the potential for primary ligament repair or re-attachment of ligament avulsion injuries. If exploration occurs later than 2–3 weeks after the injury scar tissue formation makes this difficult and ligament reconstruction may then be required. The outcome of ligament re-attachment is usually better than a late ligament reconstruction. However, for either treatment recovery is less reliable than following MCL injury and a return to normal function is uncommon.

Medial meniscus and lateral meniscus

The menisci are C-shaped fibrocartilaginous structures, attached at their periphery sitting between the convex femoral condyles and the relatively flat tibial surfaces. The menisci have several important functions but the primary one is to increase the area of contact between the articulating tibial and femoral surfaces. Stress is a product of load and surface area; thus, increasing the contact area reduces the articular cartilage stress. Meniscal injuries may occur in a health meniscus or as degenerate tears, which occur through abnormal meniscal tissue. Meniscal pathology is more common in an unstable knee, for example after ACL injury.

History

Injury to a normal meniscus is typically associated with a history of injury and usually occurs in young patients. The classic mechanism for this is a twisting injury upon a weight-bearing flexed knee. These injuries normally lead to localized acute pain over the joint line of the injured meniscus. The injury description is often of a relatively minor nature. A sportsperson may attempt to continue playing and is often able fully bear weight. This contrasts with the immediate loss of function in other significant sports -related ligament injuries, for example ACL rupture.

Degenerate meniscal tears normally occur in patients older than 35 years. Because the meniscus is abnormal it is susceptible to injury and may develop a tear with innocuous trauma that the patient may not recognize as an injury. These tears may be asymptomatic but when associated with symptoms typically cause pain that is exacerbated by activity and by twisting activities in particular. Patients with degenerate meniscal tears may also note an effusion.

Examination

The menisci are relatively avascular with blood vessels penetrating only the periphery of the meniscus via their attachments. Significant bleeding into the joint is rare and only occurs with very peripheral tears so swelling is usually of gradual onset due to a reactive synovitis.

Patients with meniscal tears typically present with signs of well-localized joint-line tenderness over the site of the meniscal tear and an effusion. A small number will present with mechanical symptoms due to entrapment of a torn meniscal fragment. This will typically be described as a catching or locking sensation.

Treatment

In younger patients with a meniscal tear through normal meniscal tissue an arthroscopic partial resection of the torn meniscus (menisectomy) or meniscal repair is usually required. During arthroscopic menisectomy the aim is to remove the minimal amount of meniscal tissue to resolve symptoms in an attempt to preserve meniscal function. Whenever possible meniscal repair is preferred to menisectomy. Evidence suggests that early meniscal repair improves the rate of meniscal preservation; therefore, an early specialist opinion is advised. For patients with a 'locked knee' urgent referral is advised. The poor vascularity of the menisci means that repair is normally only possible for peripheral tears that occur within the vascular portion of the meniscus. The healing rate of these tears is approximately 70%. Following a failed meniscal repair a proportion of patients will require further surgery, usually a partial menisectomy.

In older patients plain radiographs are important to exclude osteoarthritis, which may cause symptoms of a similar nature. The symptoms of a degenerate meniscal tear may settle spontaneously with time but for those who do not arthroscopic menisectomy is usually associated with an excellent outcome.

Patellar dislocation

Dislocation of the patella (kneecap) is a relatively common injury and always occurs laterally (Figure 10.7). Following recovery from a

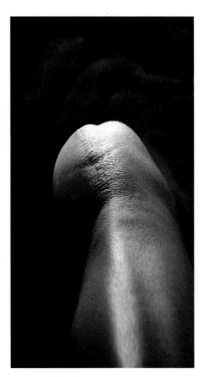

Figure 10.7 Patellar dislocation.

first-time dislocation the medial soft tissue restraints are weakened and as a result less force is required to cause subsequent dislocation. As a consequence after an initial dislocation recurrence is very common.

It is estimated that in up to 90% of patients there are predisposing factors leading to patellar dislocation. These include generalized ligament laxity, tibial or femoral malrotation, genu valgum (knock-knees) and anatomical abnormalities of the patellofemoral joint itself. Patellofemoral joint abnormalities are developmental and often have a genetic basis. This dysplasia may include a combination of a poorly developed trochleal groove of the distal anterior femur, or a small or high-riding patella.

History

Following patellar dislocation patients will usually present with an acutely swollen and painful knee. Many patients will be aware of a definite patellar dislocation but those less certain of their diagnosis typically describe a history of a twisting injury associated with sudden pain and a sensation of abnormal knee movement. The history may mimic that associated with rupture of the ACL and careful examination is required to differentiate between these conditions.

Examination

After acute dislocation a haemarthrosis is usual and pain and tenderness are centred over the damaged medial soft tissues. Point tenderness may be noted at the site of the adductor tubercle. This lies in close proximity to the medial epicondyle and is the origin of one of the primary patellar restraints known as the medial patellofemoral ligament. The patella apprehension test is a useful test that involves gently applying a lateral force to the patella with the knee help in approximately 20° of flexion. Patients with an unstable patella will try to resist this motion often by externally rotating the hip and at the same time express anxiety that the patella may dislocate. This is noted as a positive patella apprehension sign.

Treatment

As with any joint dislocation, immediate management involves reducing the patella if it remains dislocated. This should be performed by extending the knee and if necessary pushing the patella medially. Radiographs should be performed to ensure there is no associated fracture, which may require urgent treatment.

The management of an uncomplicated patellar dislocation should encourage early functional recovery. There is little evidence that joint immobilization reduces the risk of further dislocation. Management of the swelling, early joint mobilization and physiotherapy should be advised. For the majority of patients sustaining a patellar dislocation most non-operative treatment provides the basis of management; however, these patients are prone to chronic patellofemoral pain. For patients who experience recurrent patellar dislocation referral to a specialist may be considered as there are operative procedures that successfully restore stability to the patellofemoral joint.

Further reading

Baker BS. Meniscus injuries. http://emedicine.medscape.com/article/90661-overview (accessed 15 December 2015)

Brukner P, Khan K. *Clinical sports medicine*, 4th edn. McGraw-Hill Australia, 2012.

DeBerardino TM. Medial collateral knee ligament injury. http://emedicine.medscape.com/article/89890-overview (accessed 15 December 2015)

Gammons M, Sherwin SW. Anterior cruciate ligament injury. http://emedicine.medscape.com/article/89442-overview (accessed 15 December 2015).

McRae R. *Pocket book of orthopaedics and fractures*, 2nd edn. Churchill Livingstone, London, 2006.

Millar M, Thompson S. *DeLee & Drez's orthopaedic sports medicine*, 4th edn. Saunders, 2014.

Wardrope J, English B. *Musculo-skeletal problems in emergency medicine*. Oxford University Press, Oxford, 1998.

CHAPTER 11

Non-traumatic Knee Problems

Jim Wardrope[1] *and Paul M. Sutton*[2]

[1]Northern General Hospital, Sheffield, UK
[2]Sheffield Orthopaedics Ltd, Sheffield, UK

OVERVIEW

- This chapter outlines the history and examination of the patient with non-traumatic knee pain.
- It describes the management of anterior knee pain, bursitis around the knee, extensor mechanism problems and non-traumatic swollen knee.

Anterior knee pain

Anterior knee pain is a very common condition. The patellofemoral joint transmits up to three times a person's body weight when going up stairs (Figure 11.1) and up to eight times body weight in rising from the squatting position. The common causes of anterior knee pain are outlined in Box 11.1.

Osgood–Schlatter disease is inflammation with or without fragmentation of the apophysis of the tibial tuberosity. It occurs in adolescents and is probably overdiagnosed and cannot occur after skeletal maturity. *Tendinopathy* may occur at the patellar insertions of the quadriceps and patellar tendons. Very rarely a bipartite patella can give rise to pain due to inflammation of the cartilaginous connection (Figure 11.2).

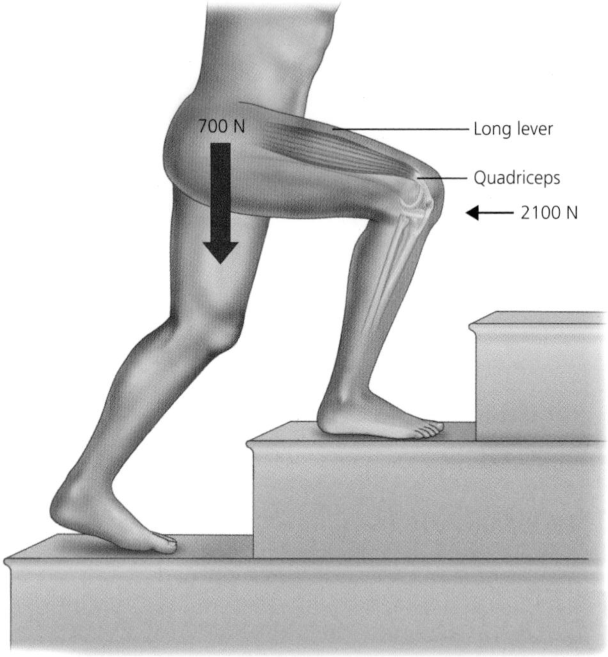

History

The history is of pain in the anterior knee on exercise. The pain is exacerbated by activities that load the extensor mechanism or patellofemoral joint such as walking up stairs or squatting. There is no history of trauma. There may be a sensation of instability or functional giving way. The condition is often bilateral. Tendinopathy is common in sportspeople, especially where jumping is involved. Tendinopathy is usually associated with very well-localized pain and tenderness. Obesity is known to predispose to patellofemoral pain and osteoarthritis.

Examination

Examine the hip when the patient complains of knee pain, especially when there are no objective signs of knee pathology such as swelling.

ABC of Common Soft Tissue Disorders, First Edition.
Edited by Francis Morris, Jim Wardrope and Paul Hattam.
© 2016 John Wiley & Sons, Ltd. Published 2016 by John Wiley & Sons, Ltd.

Figure 11.1 The knee is subject to large forces; for example, simply going up stairs results in three times the body weight going through the patellofemoral joint.

Box 11.1 **Common causes of anterior knee pain**

Patellofemoral syndrome (sometimes termed chondromalacia patella)
Patellar or quadriceps tendinopathy
Entheseiopathy
Patellofemoral osteoarthritis
Osgood–Schlatter disease

Slipped upper femoral epiphysis and fracture of the neck of femur may present only with knee pain. Failure to think of hip pathology may lead to important delays to treatment.

With patellofemoral syndrome there will be little to find on examination. There may be signs of patellar misalignment or quadriceps wasting (especially vastus medialis). With tendinopathies careful

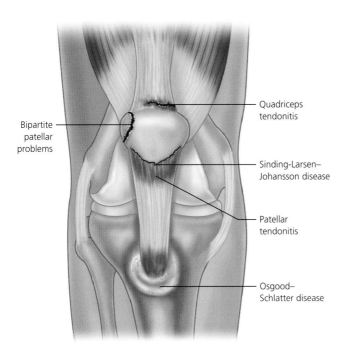

Figure 11.2 Showing sites of quadriceps insertion entheseiopathy, bipartite patella problems, Sinding-Larsen–Johansson disease, patellar tendinitis and Osgood–Schlatter disease.

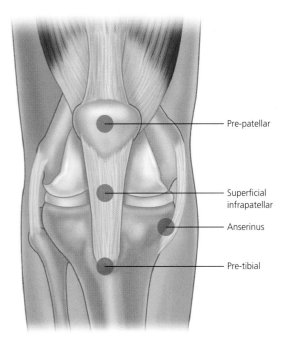

Figure 11.3 Positions of knee bursae.

palpation should localize the problem to the tendon or one of the tendon insertions. There is usually full range of movement. Resisted extension may be painful in tendinopathies and with the entheseiopathies.

Differential diagnosis

Exclude hip pathology.

Investigations are seldom helpful but plain x-rays are indicated if the pain has been present for more than 6 weeks or if there are red-flag symptoms such as night pain or bony swelling. Ultrasound or magnetic resonance imaging (MRI) may be indicated if there is a suggestion of a tendon tear or tendinopathy.

The diagnosis will be suggested by the age of the patient and clinical findings. In young women patellar tracking problems are common. In athletes tendinopathy is common. In the middle-aged or older patient osteoarthritis is more likely. Rarely, tumour or osteochondritis dessicans may present with anterior knee pain hence the need to obtain x-rays if the symptoms are prolonged or if red-flag symptoms are present.

Treatment

The treatment will depend on the diagnosis but almost all these conditions are improved by physiotherapy. This may mean correction of muscle imbalance, stretching, taping, orthotics or functional bracing. Tendinopathies should be treated with an eccentric exercise programme. Many physiotherapy interventions including eccentric exercises are easily taught and can be used as a self-help programme.

Bursitis

Introduction

Bursitis is a common condition. Pre-patellar and infrapatellar bursitis are common in those who have to kneel a lot in their work such as carpet fitters and plumbers. Gout is another common precipitant. A blow to the front of the knee may cause acute bleeding into the bursa or may lead to inflammation. A penetrating injury should heighten the suspicion for a septic bursitis. See Figure 11.3.

Pes anserinus bursitis occurs is the bursa on the upper medial tibia where the tendons of sartorius, gracilis and semitendinosus glide over the tibial attachment of the medial collateral ligament. It is common in patients with osteoarthritis and obesity due to abnormal loading. It may be secondary to hamstring tightness. It is more common in patients with diabetes.

Clinical features

The history is one of non-traumatic swelling and pain in the pre-patellar area or over the tibial tuberosity. There is often erythaema and increased heat around the area, with localized swelling and tenderness over the bursa. There is no knee effusion. Passive knee movements in the range 0–90° are usually relatively pain-free. With higher degrees of flexion the bursa may become compressed, leading to pain.

In pes anserinus bursitis the pain is localized to the medial side of tibia at the site of knee. Erythema and heat are uncommon but there may be swelling.

Investigations are not normally required unless there is a history of blunt or penetrating trauma when plain x-ray is required to exclude bony injury or a foreign body. If there is marked tenderness over the medial tibial area then a stress fracture needs to be excluded. If symptoms are prolonged x-ray is indicated.

Differential diagnosis

These conditions are often very painful with florid signs of local inflammation. At times the clinician may be concerned about the possibility of septic arthritis of the knee. However, the swellings are anterior and extra-articular so there will be no knee effusion. Unlike a septic arthritis, movements in the range 0–90° should be relatively pain-free.

Most bursitis is inflammatory but septic bursitis is not uncommon, especially where there is a history of penetrating injury.

Treatment

Non-steroidal anti-inflammatory drugs (NSAIDs), rest and avoidance of kneeling are the initial treatments. Antibiotics may be indicated if sepsis is suspected. Most of the acute signs of inflammation settle within 5–7 days but the swelling is often persistent, sometimes taking several months to resolve.

Surgical drainage may be required if an abscess is forming. Drainage may result in a sinus that might take months to heal.

Pes anserinus bursitis is a self-limiting condition. Rest, topical NSAIDs and occasionally physiotherapy may be of benefit.

Quadriceps tendon rupture/patellar tendon rupture

Introduction

These injuries require timely diagnosis and, usually, surgical repair. The mechanism is forced flexion while the quadriceps is contracting or an explosive extension force as in high jumping. Quadriceps tendon tears are more common in the elderly and patellar tendon tears are typically seen in younger, active individuals.

Clinical features

The patient is typically unable to weight bear and will complain the knee feels very weak and unstable. There will swelling over the anterior aspect of the knee. On palpation there will be tenderness and a gap may be felt. The patient will be unable to straight leg raise but a more subtle sign is that with quadriceps activation there will be no movement of the patella.

X-rays are required to exclude bone injury to the patella or tibial tuberosity. Figure 11.4 shows a high-riding patella in a case of patellar tendon rupture. If the diagnosis is unclear ultrasound or MRI may be indicated.

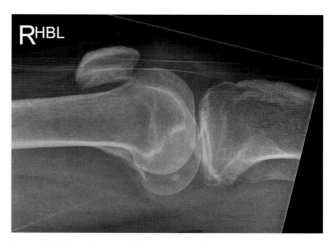

Figure 11.4 High riding patella in case of patellar tendon rupture.

Treatment

Patients suspected of having these injuries should be referred promptly to an orthopaedic service for surgical repair.

Non-traumatic swollen knee

Introduction

This is a very common presentation. Usually the patient is older. A non-traumatic knee effusion in a younger person is unusual. The causes of knee swelling are listed in Table 11.1.

Clinical features

In the younger patient a detailed medical history and general examination will be important. In the absence of trauma, a knee swelling is more likely to be due to significant pathology. Ask about other joint problems, systemic symptoms such as chills, fevers or loss of appetite, family history and bleeding problems. In adolescents a sexual history may be required. Check temperature, examine for rashes, check lymph nodes and check other joints, especially the hands. On knee examination erythema and local heat are important signs. Establish whether the swelling is due to an effusion, pre-patellar swelling or bony swelling.

Investigation

X-rays are often unhelpful but are indicated in the young to exclude osteochondritis dessicans or tumour. In the older patient the yield

Table 11.1 Causes of non-traumatic knee swelling.

Young	Adult	Older
Trauma	Trauma	Osteoarthritis
Juvenile rheumatoid	Gout	Degenerative meniscal disease
Osteochondritis dissecans	Degenerative meniscal disease	Gout/pseudogout
Other arthritides	Rheumatoid	Anticoagulant-induced haemarthrosis
Sepsis	Other arthritides	Sepsis
Tumour	Sepsis	Tumour
Reiter's syndrome	Tumour	
Coagulopathy-induced haemarthrosis		

of positive findings is small but they are indicated if there are symptoms of true locking, a history of a loose body or red-flag symptoms are such as night, prolonged or worsening pain.

Joint aspiration is indicated if there are signs of sepsis, either local or systemic. If the effusion has occurred suddenly then haemarthrosis should be suspected and this would be an indication for aspiration. The aspirate should be sent for an immediate Gram stain, culture, sensitivity and microscopy for crystals. A negative Gram stain does not exclude septic arthritis.

Differential diagnosis

The range of diagnosis is wide and summarized in Table 11.1. In the young and in the absence of trauma a joint effusion is usually significant and warrants careful investigation. In the older patient degenerative disease is an extremely common cause and in the absence of any red-flag symptoms or signs investigation may be deferred until simple treatments have had a chance to take effect.

Treatment

Treatment will depend entirely on the cause. Have a low threshold for referral of a young patient for a further opinion and investigation.

Acute gout and pseudogout are treated with NSAIDs or colchicine. If these are contraindicated then a short dose of prednisolone is usually curative. Longer-term treatment can be with allopurinol.

Osteoarthritis is treated according to symptoms. Mild-to-moderate symptoms may be managed with anti-inflammatory drugs (local may be effective), graded exercise and weight reduction. More severe symptoms may require an orthopaedic surgical opinion.

Most of the other diagnoses will require specialist referral.

Further reading

Brukner P, Khan K. *Clinical sports medicine*, 4th edn. McGraw-Hill Australia, 2012.

Brukner P, Khan K. Bursae and bursitis of the knee. Wheeless' Textbook of Orthopaedics. http://www.wheelessonline.com/ortho/bursae_and_bursitis_of_the_knee (accessed 15 December 2015).

McRae R. *Pocket book of orthopaedics and fractures*, 2nd edn. Churchill Livingstone, London, 2006.

Millar M, Thompson S. *DeLee & Drez's orthopaedic sports medicine*, 4th edn. Saunders, 2014.

Wardrope J, English B. *Musculo-skeletal problems in emergency medicine*. Oxford University Press, Oxford, 1998.

CHAPTER 12

Calf and Shin Problems

Roger Dalton[1], Mark B. Davies[2] and Ashley Jones[1]

[1]Chesterfield FC, Chesterfield, UK
[2]Sheffield Teaching Hospitals NHS Foundation Trust, Sheffield, UK

OVERVIEW

- The lower leg is prone to various types of musculoskeletal inflammation, which cause pain and swelling of the calf.

- People who engage in sporting activity are particularly at risk of significant injuries to the lower leg and calf.

- A careful history and examination is vital in order to determine the cause of the symptoms and to differentiate musculoskeletal injuries from non-traumatic conditions such as deep venous thrombosis.

- Modification of gait using orthotic shoe implants may be a useful treatment strategy.

- More advanced treatments such as electromagnetic field therapy, ultrasound therapy, iontophoresis and phonophoresis have no clear evidence base supporting their use.

Introduction

The lower leg contains bones, muscles, tendons, nerves, blood vessels and connective tissue. Injury to or overuse of these structures can manifest as calf and/or shin pain. This chapter will outline the more common musculoskeletal complaints.

Muscular injury

The main muscles in the lower leg are divided into anterior and posterior groups. Figure 12.1 shows the anatomical relationships of the anterior and posterior groups.

Musculotendinous injuries are the most common cause of pain in the lower leg and the medial belly of the gastrocnemius muscle is the commonest site of injury. The lateral belly of gastrocnemius, the more distal gastrocnemius bulk and the soleus muscle can also be injured, though less frequently. These injuries and their effects may be clinically obvious, such as the football player who feels a sharp sudden pain in the calf when running with the ball; however, more indolent presentations can be more problematic to the clinician. The soleus muscle is less commonly injured than the gastrocnemius, and is prone to more occult presentation with calf 'tightness', as it often

becomes hardened when overstretched, resulting in an inflexible portion of muscle that is prone to injury.

The examination of a patient with a musculotendinous injury should follow the 'look/feel/move' sequence. The patient's gait should be noted, whether antalgic or normal. Observation of the site of injury may reveal a clear defect in the muscle/tendon and erythema may be present, although this is unusual.

On palpation, the skin over the site of injury may be warm to touch.

Local tenderness will be present when palpated and a defect may be felt in patients with a severe (grade 3) muscular tear (see Table 12.1).

Assessment of movement is vital in calf injuries. Active, passive and resisted movements of the ankle and knee should be noted. In most cases, active and resisted plantar flexion of the foot will reproduce the pain. The functional status of the muscle can be assessed by observing the patient performing a heel raise. A minor muscle injury will result in some pain when performing a heel raise, whereas a more significant injury may prevent the patient from being able to complete this movement.

Following any muscular trauma, cryotherapy and compression are the most useful forms of treatment. These counteract the effect of high levels of vasoactive chemicals that are released around the injured tissue.

If the patient has marked pain when weight bearing, crutches should be used to prevent any further damage to the connective tissue and allow the healing process to work without interruption. Heel raises in the patients shoes may be useful to reduce the stress put upon the posterior lower limb structures.

Once the early inflammatory symptoms have subsided and the patient is fully weight bearing, simple concentric strengthening such as simple calf raises can occur. The gastrocnemius and soleus muscles should be targeted. It is also important that the patient is educated on stretching techniques for the surrounding muscular structures to prevent muscular tightness and help to avoid secondary injuries.

Achilles injuries/tendinopathy

The Achilles tendon is formed from the distal tendinous portions of the gastrocnemius and soleus muscles. It inserts into the

ABC of Common Soft Tissue Disorders, First Edition.
Edited by Francis Morris, Jim Wardrope and Paul Hattam.
© 2016 John Wiley & Sons, Ltd. Published 2016 by John Wiley & Sons, Ltd.

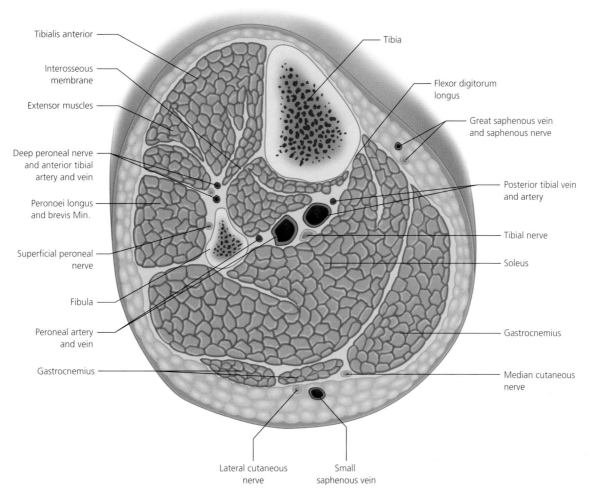

Figure 12.1 Calf anatomy, and the anatomical relationships of the anterior and posterior groups.

Table 12.1 Functional grading of muscular injuries of the calf (after Brukner and Khan 2006).

Grade	Symptoms	Signs
1	Some acute pain, more painful after activity	Tenderness on palpation, no functional disability, but painful resisted movements
2	Marked immediate pain, worsening over 12–24 hours	Tenderness on palpation, minor functional disability, but painful active and resisted movements Bruising may be evident
3	Immediate severe pain, which may decrease with time	Tenderness on palpation, significant functional disability Painful passive, active and resisted movements Bruising likely

posterior aspect of the calcaneum, with a bursa situated between the calcaneum and the tendon. It is a wide, strong tendon, but can be damaged in a number of ways.

Achilles tendinopathy

Achilles tendinopathy often results from overuse of the tendon. Equally, tendinopathy happens in very overweight, sedentary patients because of the large forces from excessive body weight overloading the Achilles tendon. In either patient group, this results in a localized inflammatory process causing swelling, pain and stiffness. Several specific factors contribute to the development of Achilles tendinopathy. Undertaking certain types of exercise or sport (squash) with poorly developed calf muscles leads to overloading of the tendon. Similarly, rapid increases in training (e.g. hill running/sprinting) can contribute to tendon overload. Inadequately supported footwear and flat-footedness also contribute to tendinopathy as they cause overstretching of the tendon. Microtears in the tendon fibres result in inflammation coupled with the tendon's poor blood supply, lead to pain, chronic scarring

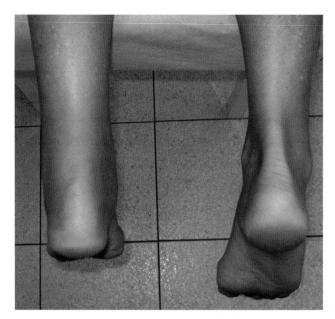

Figure 12.2 Simmond's test. When the right calf (unaffected) is squeezed, the foot plantar-flexes. When the left calf is squeezed, the foot does not move due to the left Achilles tendon being ruptured. Note the loss of tendon definition on the left due to swelling.

and intratendinous degeneration. The patient will complain of pain and stiffness, often worse in the morning (start-up pain). The pain often eases with gentle exercise, but will recur thereafter. On examination, the patient will have tenderness over the Achilles tendon and crepitus may be present in severe cases where the surrounding paratenon is inflamed. The tendon may be palpably thicker than an unaffected tendon with a classic fusiform, midsubstance swelling. Active and passive plantar flexion will be relatively comfortable for the patient, but resisted movements will cause pain, due to the increased loading of the tendon.

Simple cases of Achilles tendinopathy can be treated with rest, anti-inflammatory medication and eccentric exercises directed by a physiotherapist.

Heel raises in footwear can be useful, especially in sports-related tendonitis. Dry needling techniques, injections of high-volume fluids into the paratenon, platelet-rich plasma injections and extracorporeal shockwave treatments have been tried with some success. Steroid injections should never be undertaken to avoid the risk of tendon rupture. Surgery can have a role in recalcitrant cases.

Of paramount importance is to distinguish Achilles tendinopathy from a ruptured tendon. Patients with Achilles tendon tears classically complain of sudden pain at the posterior aspect of the ankle. Many patients feel that they have been kicked on the ankle, or hit with an object, such as a hockey ball. The patient will be unable to walk normally and often display evidence of loss of tiptoe or propulsive power. Plantar flexion of the foot may still be possible due to the function of the long toe flexors and the peroneus muscles. On examination, the patient will have swelling and tenderness over the posterior aspect of the ankle. There may be a palpable gap in the tendon, although this is not always present.

The integrity (or otherwise) of the Achilles tendon can be clinically assessed using the Simmond's test, sometimes referred to as the 'calf squeeze test'. The patient kneels on a raised surface, for example an examination couch (Figure 12.2). The calf of the unaffected limb will, when squeezed, produce plantar flexion of the foot, due to the contraction of the gastrocnemius muscle and the subsequent 'drawing up' of the Achilles tendon. If the tendon is not intact, plantar flexion will not occur, as the ruptured tendon cannot act as a pulley to move the foot.

Tendon rupture can be confirmed by ultrasound or magnetic resonance imaging (MRI) examination of the tendon. Plain radiographs do not visualize the tendon; however, they are indicated to identify small avulsion fractures that may occur. The patient should be immobilized in a plaster cast, with the foot plantar-flexed in an equinus position and referred to an orthopaedic surgeon for ongoing management.

Treatment of Achilles rupture

Treatment of these injuries can be surgical or non-surgical, dependent on the patient's circumstances. There is a slightly higher rate of re-rupture of the tendon in those patients managed non-operatively. In cases treated surgically, the lower re-rupture rate has to be weighed against the post-operative complications of wound infection and iatrogenic sural nerve injury. Relative contraindications to surgery include factors that may inhibit tendon and soft tissue healing such as diabetes, steroid therapy and peripheral vascular disease. In these cases, non-operative management is recommended.

With ultrasonographic assessment, in those cases where the tendon ends can be well apposed with the foot in 20° of plantar flexion, current evidence seems to support that these patients can be managed non-operatively in a functional brace provided that the tendon ends do not displace over a 6-week period. In those patients with unapposable tendon ends or those with delayed presentations, surgical apposition of the tendon ends is advocated followed by rehabilitation in a functional brace. All cases need physiotherapy input to optimize outcome.

Physiotherapy focuses on returning the patient to their pre-injury state of mobility. This requires re-education of the surrounding musculature and mobilization of the ankle joint. Calf muscle massage is indicated, as a degree of muscle tightness will be present following immobilization. Friction massage to the damaged tendon increases blood flow and improves scar tissue elasticity.

Early active exercises using a resistance band should be used to treat muscle atrophy, progressing to full weight-bearing exercises once a full range of movement has been achieved.

Shin splints

The term 'shin splints' refers to a spectrum of symptoms and causative pathologies that cause lower leg pain and functional limitations, which can be significant, especially for the elite athlete. The underlying cause(s) can be divided into soft tissue and bony pathologies.

Non-bony pathologies

Medial tibial stress syndrome (MTSS) is a collective term for lower leg pain. It encompasses over-tightness of lower leg muscles, including soleus, gastrocnemius and the plantar flexors. The resulting stresses cause a reduced ability to absorb impact such as those caused by running, which, when combined with the accompanying reduction in tibial remodelling ability, leads to tibial bowing and excessive muscle fatigue. This causes pain and impaired function. MTSS can occur in isolation, or can progress to stress fractures and/or chronic compartment syndrome.

Predisposing factors include having flat feet and over-pronation when running. Runners and dancers are particularly prone to MTSS, which should be suspected if they present with lower leg pain.

Patients with MTSS characteristically give a history of indolent pain, which worsens with exercise and eases when resting. However, the pain can occasionally ease with exercise and may be present at rest.

Examination findings are often non-specific. Tenderness along the lateral tibial border may be present and resisted ankle movements may cause replication of symptoms. Neurological and vascular examination is invariably normal, although if patients with chronic compartment syndrome are examined after exercising, neurological findings may be present.

Radiographs are indicated to exclude alternative pathology such as fractures or tumours, although MTSS itself has no specific radiographic features. MRI scanning may reveal periosteal oedema, marrow oedema and fractures.

Treatment of MTSS/shin splints

It is important to rest the injured limb, as this allows the damaged tissue to recover and remodel. This is acceptable for the majority of patients, but can be problematic in the professional sportsperson. A number of more specific treatments have been tried to manage MTSS including stretching exercises, ice massage, leg braces, electromagnetic field therapy, ultrasound therapy, iontophoresis and phonophoresis. There is little definitive evidence that any of these treatments are effective, although extracorporeal shockwave therapy appears to have the most promise.

MTSS commonly causes underdevelopment of tibialis anterior and soleus and a specific strengthening regime for these muscles may be appropriate. Deep tissue massage may also improve symptoms, particularly working on tight areas of muscle that may otherwise reduce the range of movement at the ankle. Active ankle mobilization may be helpful if a reduced range of movement is present.

Common peroneal nerve injury

The peroneal nerve arises from the sciatic nerve. It supplies sensation to the anterior and lateral leg and to the dorsum of the foot and dorsi-flexes the foot at the ankle.

Traumatic injuries to the common peroneal nerve can result from fibular head fractures causing 'foot drop' due to the inability of the patient to dorsi-flex the foot. It can also be caused by 'peroneal strike', a technique used in martial arts and in law enforcement, where the leg is struck just above the knee on the posterior surface. This produces temporary foot drop and painful paraesthesia, which can be incapacitating for the victim.

Non-traumatic peroneal neuropathy can occur in a number of situations, including prolonged bed rest and prolonged positioning in obstetric stirrups, again causing foot drop and paraesthesia.

Baker's cyst

A Baker's cyst is a benign swelling of a synovial bursa, often the semimembranous bursa, and may occur secondary to a degenerate meniscal tear. It causes swelling in the popliteal fossa and, although usually asymptomatic, causes calf pain, swelling and redness that may mimic a deep venous thrombosis or thrombophlebitis if ruptured. A patient with a Baker's cyst will have a palpable swelling in the popliteal fossa, often palpated most easily with the knee slightly flexed. If the cyst ruptures, pain is felt behind the knee and the resulting drainage of synovial fluid distally causes calf swelling, pain and erythema. It is important to distinguish a Baker's cyst from a popliteal aneurysm in patients presenting with popliteal swelling and to investigate patients with painful lower leg swelling for the possibility of deep venous thrombosis.

Bony pathologies

The tibia and fibula are prone to stress damage, which can manifest as bony inflammation (osteitis), periosteal inflammation and stress fractures. Contributing factors include altered gait (e.g. over pronation), over training, excessive running on hard surfaces (e.g. road running), exercise that is disproportionate to fitness levels and

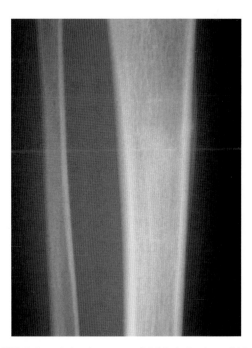

Figure 12.3 Periosteal elevation over medial tibia, indicating a tibial stress fracture.

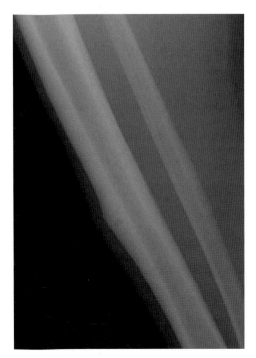

Figure 12.4 Tibial stress fracture with cortical infraction.

previous injuries. Inflammation of the bone surface occurs, resulting in periosteitis and/or osteitis. Microfractures can occur and, if untreated, the body's ability to remodel these microfractures is impaired. The microfractures then propagate leading to a complete fracture line.

The history given by patients with bone pathology will be of reasonably well-localized pain which is worse with exercise, although, in some cases, the pain can be severe when starting to exercise, ease somewhat as exercising continues and then worsen again. This pattern is often seen in runners, who feel they can 'run the pain off' only for it to worsen with time. Acute worsening of symptoms can indicate that a fracture has become complete; that is, the cortex has become completely separated.

On examination the skin overlying the fracture may be warmer than surrounding skin, especially if the fracture site is relatively superficial. Bony tenderness may be present and the fracture site will be painful when vibratory forces are applied, for example percussing the affected area or applying a tuning fork to the skin overlying the fracture.

Plain radiographs can be useful in the diagnosis of a stress fracture. Periosteal elevation can be seen in some cases, but will not be evident until 2–3 weeks after symptoms start (Figure 12.3). Radiographs may also reveal visible cortical infractions (Figure 12.4).

Further reading

Allen M. Overview of exercise induced lower leg pain. *Br J Sports Med* 2011;**45**:2 e2.
Batt M. Medial tibial stress syndrome. *Br J Sports Med* 2011;**45**:2 e2.
Brukner P, Khan K. *Clinical sports medicine*, 3rd edn. McGraw-Hill Professional, 2006.

CHAPTER 13

Soft Tissue Injuries of the Ankle

Hasan Qayyum[1], Chris M. Blundell[2] and Joanna Ollerenshaw[1]

[1]Sheffield Teaching Hospitals NHS Foundation Trust, Sheffield, UK
[2]Claremont Private Hospital, Sheffield, UK

OVERVIEW

- Injuries to the ankle are a common presentation to emergency departments and primary care services.
- A correct diagnosis requires a good history including mechanism of injury and an examination supported with stability tests.
- The Ottawa Ankle Rules reduce the need of imaging by up to 40%.
- High ankle sprains account for 10–15% of all ankle sprains, often caused by a forced external rotation mechanism. They often have a delayed diagnosis. Patients present with pain above the tibial plafond with x-rays often being normal.
- Treating soft tissue injuries of the ankle classically involves the PRICE approach of protection, rest, ice, compression and elevation as most of these injuries present in the acute phase. Analgesia, preferably a non-steroidal anti-inflammatory drug, will help alleviate pain and swelling. An early referral to physiotherapy is strongly recommended.

Soft tissue injuries of the ankle often cause problems for people across all walks of life. Be it a mechanical fall causing the ankle to twist, or forced external rotation and hyperflexion from collision sports, a sprained ankle causes debilitating symptoms including the inability to weight bear.

Although, more common in young adults and children, these injuries are increasingly being recognized in older people, probably due to the increased levels of recreational activity in this age group. Nearly half of acute soft tissue injuries to the ankle result from direct collisions in sports such as basketball and football (Garrick and Requa 1988).

Anatomy of the ankle joint

The ankle joint is a complex hinge joint allowing dorsiflexion (extension) and plantar flexion (flexion) and is formed by the articulation of the distal tibia, distal fibula and talus (see Figure 13.1).

Ankle joint ligaments can be considered in two groups: the lateral and medial ligament complexes.

Lateral ligament complex

The lateral ligament complex is the most important ligament group, and consists of three ligaments, as follows.

1 Anterior talofibular ligament (ATFL): the most common ligament to be injured in ankle sprains (Anderson 1996, Rubin and Sallis 1996, Marder 1995, Simon 1994), the ATFL joins the anterior part of the lateral malleolus to the talus.
2 Posterior talofibular ligament (PTFL): joins the posterior part of the lateral malleolus to the talus.
3 Calcaneofibular ligament (CFL): joins the lateral malleolus to the calcaneus without attaching to the talus.

The lateral ligament complex is thin and unyielding, making it prone to injuries.

Medial ligament complex

The medial ligament complex (deltoid ligament) consists of two layers of strong, fanned fibres from the medial malleolus with the deep part attaching distally to the talus and the superficial part to the calcaneus.

Tibiofibular syndesmosis

The joint between distal fibula and the distal tibia is not a synovial joint but is part of the ankle joint complex. Injuries to this area, called high ankle sprains, are becoming increasingly diagnosed. Anterior and posterior inferior tibiofibular ligaments, and the interosseous membrane, form the stabilizers of this syndesmotic joint.

Clinical assessment of the ankle joint

Before examining an ankle joint, always spend time focusing on the precise mechanism of injury. The following history should be sought.

- Chronology of events: when did the injury occur? Was ice or a splint immediately applied?

ABC of Common Soft Tissue Disorders, First Edition.
Edited by Francis Morris, Jim Wardrope and Paul Hattam.
© 2016 John Wiley & Sons, Ltd. Published 2016 by John Wiley & Sons, Ltd.

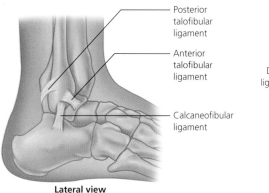
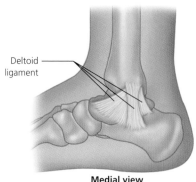

Figure 13.1 The ankle joint with supporting ligaments.

- Mechanism of injury: this could include force of collision, inversion or eversion injury.
- Weight bearing: was the patient able to walk four steps immediately after the injury?
- Were any rotational stresses applied? This is a risk factor for a high ankle sprain and a fracture.
- A previous history of ankle injuries and an assessment of the post-injury rehabilitation (Rubin and Sallis 1996, Marder 1995).
- Comorbidities like osteoporosis, osteoarthritis, rheumatoid arthritis, diabetes and peripheral vascular disease should be sought.
- A history of inflammatory symptoms like fever, chills and rigors should be elicited in the negative history. If present, rethink your differentials, considering a septic arthritis or gout.

  Note:

- high-energy injuries cause more damage,
- pay attention to the deforming direction,
- look out for bruising and swelling: they indicate more severe injuries.

Examining an ankle joint should be simple yet systematic, and should include inspection, palpation, joint movements, special tests, neurovascular status and a quick assessment of the joint above and below.

Follow a look, feel, move approach and start by looking at the patient's gait. Compare the injured ankle with the opposite side as a baseline to assess callosities, swelling, deformities and range of movement. A non-weight-bearing limb should be carefully examined for tenderness, so as to avoid blanket imaging of a whole limb. Remember, the inability to take four steps on the injured ankle is a red-flag sign and should warrant imaging.

Palpate for tenderness to the posterior edge of the medial and lateral malleoli, base of the fifth metatarsal, navicular bone and calcaneum. Also, palpate the gastrocnemius belly and check the integrity of the Achilles tendon by Simmond's squeeze test.

Always palpate the entire length of the tibia and fibula. An assessment of the knee joint and foot is mandatory to avoid missing associated injuries, for example in Maisonneuve fractures where a syndesmotic ankle injury is associated with a proximal fibula fracture.

Neurovascular integrity should be checked by palpating the posterior tibial artery (the main blood supply to the ankle) and the dorsalis pedis artery, the latter being absent in 10% of the population.

There are several special tests for assessing soft tissues supporting the ankle joint. They focus on stressing a particular ligament complex by tilting and drawing the ankle joint and looking for laxity or joint pain. These will be discussed below.

Ottawa Ankle Rules: do they work?

In brief, yes, they do. Prior to their use in emergency departments, most ankle sprains underwent radiography. Fewer than 15% of these had fractures.

Derived by the Stiell group in 1992, these clinical decision rules reduced the need for unneccessary radiographs of the ankle and foot by 30–40%. The Ottawa Ankle Rules (OARs; Figure 13.2) were subsequently validated to have a very high sensitivity of almost 100% in excluding fractures of the ankle and foot (Stiell *et al.* 1992, 1993, Bachmann *et al.* 2003).

The rules are simple to use and can be applied to any adult with an injury to the ankle, broadly defined as an area of the distal leg and the midfoot . It's worth noting that the OARs were originally designed for adult ankle injuries only. Although some validation studies have been done in children, their diagnostic accuracy in children is not comparable to adults (McConnochie *et al.* 1990, Chande 1992, Plint *et al.* 1999, Clark *et al.* 2003).

OARs state that an ankle x-ray is only required if there is pain in the malleolar zone *plus*:

- bone tenderness at posterior edge or tip of the lateral malleolus, *or*
- bone tenderness at posterior edge or tip of the medial malleolus, *or*
- inability to weight bear both immediately and in the emergency department.

OARs also recommend a foot x-ray if there is midfoot pain, *plus*:

- bone tenderness at base of the fifth metatarsal, *or*
- bone tenderness at navicular, *or*
- inability to weight bear both immediately and in the emergency department.

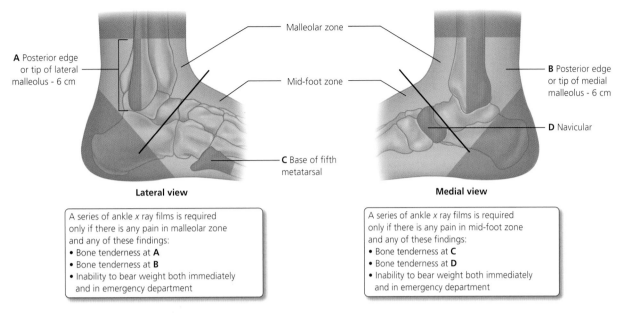

Figure 13.2 Ottawa ankle rules. Source: Bachmann *et al*. (2003). Reproduced with permission of BMJ.

Lateral ligament complex injuries

Sprains of the lateral ankle are common and minor compared to the medial ligament complex. They usually result from an inversion injury to the ankle. Some may also occur with plantar flexion as an added mechanism to inversion.

Classification

Classifying lateral ankle sprains was traditionally purely anatomical (Malliaropoulos *et al.* 2006). Ankle sprains were graded I, II or III based on the extent and severity of ligament damage, with grade I being the least and grade III being the most severe type of injury (see Table 13.1).

Recent classifications of ankle sprains have incorporated functional capacity, which includes variables such as range of motion, strength and ability to perform functional tests (De Bie *et al.* 1997).

Although both approaches have merits, they are tricky to apply when dealing with the acute ankle injury and are probably best be suited for a follow-up visit.

A more pragmatic classification suitable in the acute setting would be dividing the sprained ankle into either a stable or an unstable injury on the basis of clinical examination (Clanton and Porter 1997).

Ligament testing for lateral ligament complex injuries
Note:

- all tests best done with a relaxed patient,
- simple classification into stable or unstable will suffice,
- do not repeat tests multiple times as will hurt the patient and reduce the sensitivity of the test.

There are many clinical methods to test the stability of the lateral ankle ligaments. Perhaps the most important are the anterior drawer test and talar tilt test, which will help the examiner grade ankle sprains.

Anterior drawer test

- Indication: to test the integrity of the ATFL.
- Action: the examiner stands on the side being tested with the patient laid supine or sitting but with the knee flexed (Figure 13.3). The examiner holds the foot by cupping it at the heel in the palm of the right hand for a right injury and left hand for a left injury. The other hand stabilizes the tibia while the cupping hand firmly but slowly pulls the foot forward: anterior drawer. This draws the foot forward perpendicular to the intermalleolar axis. The test is a slow draw forward rather than a rapid snatch test: it is akin to the Lachman test at the knee.
- Positive test: anterior movement of the foot at the ankle is a positive test, sometimes associated with sulcus of the skin at the medial joint line.

Talar tilt test

- Indication: to test the integrity of ATFL and, if movement detected at the subtalar joint too, the CFL.
- Action: the examiner inverts the patient's foot, which is at neutral plantar flexion, cupping the calcaneum with one hand and using the other hand positioned over the talar dome to assess the range of talar motion (Figure 13.4).
- Positive test: increased tilting of the talus suggests a rupture of the ATFL. If the talus tilts then stops but the hindfoot continues to invert this may be coming from the subtalar joint, suggesting a CFL rupture too.

Table 13.1 Classification of ankle sprains.

Grade	Grade I	Grade II	Grade III
Function	No loss of function	Some loss of function	Near total loss of function
Laxity	No ligament laxity	Positive anterior drawer test; negative talar tilt test	Positive anterior drawer test and talar tilt test
			IIIA: anterior drawer movement of 3 mm or less on stress radiograph
			IIIB: anterior drawer movement of greater than 3 mm on stress radiograph
Bruising	Little or no bruising	Bruising	Bruising
Tenderness	No point tenderness	Point tenderness	Extreme point tenderness
Range of motion	Decreased total ankle motion to 5° or less	Decreased total ankle motion to 5–10°	Decreased total ankle motion to greater than 10°
Swelling	Swelling to 0.5 cm or less	Swelling to 0.5–2.0 cm	Swelling greater than 2.0 cm

Source: Malliaropoulos *et al.* (2006). Reproduced with permission of Elsevier.

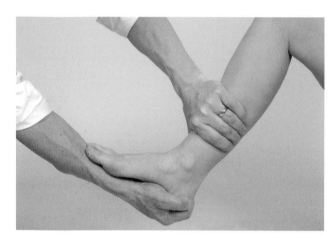

Figure 13.3 Anterior drawer test.

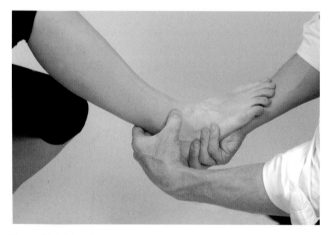

Figure 13.4 Talar tilt test.

Note: pain in the high ankle area with increased talar movements associated with apprehension as the talus rotates suggests a possible syndesmotic injury.

ATFL stress test

- Indication: to stress the ATFL to assess a grade I/II sprain.
- Action: also known as the plantar flexion test, the examiner cups the calcaneum with one hand, using the other hand wrapped around the dorsum of the foot to plantar flex and invert the ankle (Figure 13.5).
- Positive test: pain over the lateral side of the ankle.

This test is best done once the acute phase of injury has subsided. The ATFL is the most frequently injured component lateral complex ligament of the ankle. It is also the most important lateral support for the ankle. It is most frequently injured in plantar flexion and inversion. In contrast, the PTFL is the strongest ligament in the lateral complex and is injured only in extreme inversion injuries.

CFL stress test

- Indication: to stress the CFL to assess a grade I/II sprain.
- Action: also known as the inversion test, the examiner cups the calcaneum with one hand using the other hand placed over the dorsum of the foot to gently dorsiflex and varus stress the ankle (Figure 13.6).
- Positive test: pain over the lateral aspect of the ankle with or without restricted movements.

It's worth remembering that a CFL injury rarely occurs without a concurrent ATFL injury. The ATFL is stressed in plantar flexion and inversion, while the CFL is stressed in dorsiflexion and inversion. Both of these ligaments provide lateral stability to the ankle.

Medial ligament complex injuries

This strong fan-shaped ligament is the medial support of the ankle, limiting foot eversion. It is a rare ligament to injure in isolation, and is usually associated with a fracture or a tibiofibular syndesmosis injury.

On the medial side of the ankle, fractures occur around seven times more frequently than ligament injuries. This is attributed to enhanced bone and soft tissue support (Wolfe *et al.* 2001).

With medial malleolar swelling and tenderness, always suspect a Maisonneuve fracture and/or a syndesmotic injury.

Medial collateral ligament stress test

- Indication: to stress the deltoid ligament for assessing a grade I/II sprain.

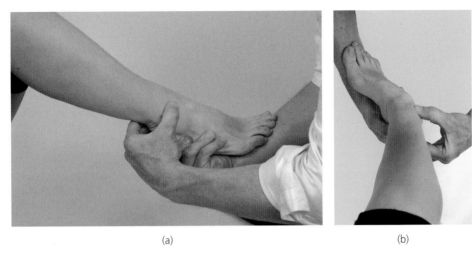

Figure 13.5 (a) The ATFL test shown with examiner cupping the calcaneum with one hand and using the other hand to plantar flex and invert the ankle. (b) Axial view of the ATFL test in application with the ankle in plantar flexion and inversion.

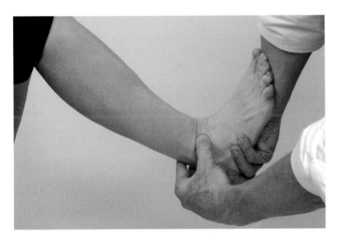

Figure 13.6 CFL stress test.

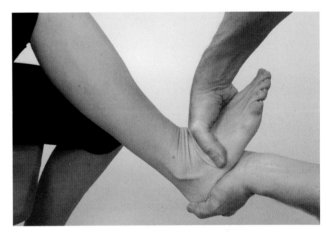

Figure 13.7 Medial collateral ligament stress test.

- Action: the examiner cups the calcaneum with one hand and dorsiflexes the ankle; with the other hand placed over the dorsum of the foot a valgus stress is applied to the ankle (Figure 13.7).
- Positive test: pain over the medial side of the ankle with or without laxity.

High (syndesmotic) ankle sprain

Commonly caused by hyperflexion and forced external rotational ankle injuries in football and downhill skiing, high ankle sprains account for 10–15% of all ankle sprains. They often have a delayed diagnosis. Patients present with pain above the tibial plafond with x-rays often being normal.

External rotation test can make a clinical diagnosis and when combined with tenderness over the syndesmosis this test is sensitive and unlikely to miss a high ankle sprain (Lamb *et al.* 2009).

External rotation stress test

- Indication: to determine injury to the tibiofibular syndesmotic ligaments.

- Action: the examiner cups the heel and externally rotates the ankle, stabilizing the knee with the other hand (Figure 13.8).
- Positive test: pain felt over the anterolateral aspect of the ankle at the level of the syndesmosis. Instability is rarely felt.

A high ankle sprain has a prolonged recovery time lasting months and missed injuries may lead to joint diastasis. Sport may have to be avoided for around 6–8 weeks. A low index of suspicion and early referral to orthopaedics should be the initial management.

Ankle instability and chronic ankle pain

Chronic ankle problems can occur in up to a third of acute lateral ligament injuries with instability and ankle pain being common chronic symptoms. This may follow a serious ankle injury or repeated minor injuries. Patients usually present with a history of persistent pain and instability, especially on uneven ground (Matharu *et al.* 2010).

Chronic ankle instability can be either functional or mechanical.

- Functional: subjective complaint commonly seen with lateral ligament injuries and thought to be due to proprioception problems.

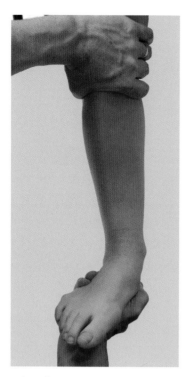

Figure 13.8 External rotation stress test.

Occult osteochondral loose bodies may get diagnosed as functional instability.

- Mechanical: due to laxity of damaged ligaments leading to increased ankle motion with stress testing.

Stress radiography has variable reliability for diagnosing chronic instability while magnetic resonance imaging (MRI) and clinical evaluation are sensitive for diagnosing chronic mechanical instability.

The treatment for chronic ankle instability is functional rehabilitation focusing on muscle strengthening and proprioception exercises. Surgical repair is reserved for cases where rehabilitation fails, typically beyond 6 months.

Treatment: interventions and rehabilitation

Treating soft tissue injuries of the ankle classically involves the PRICE approach of protection, rest, ice, compression and elevation as most of these injuries present in the acute phase. Analgesia, preferably a non-steroidal anti-inflammatory drug (NSAID), will help alleviate pain and swelling. An early referral to physiotherapy is strongly recommended.

Evidence-based treatment of ankle sprains can be divided into the following phases.

Acute/protected motion phase of rehabilitation

This is the phase in which the majority of ankle injuries present to the emergency department. Usually within the first 72 hours following injury, significant pain, swelling and partial or no weight bearing characterize this phase.

- Early weight bearing with support: the benefits of weight bearing *as tolerated* are well documented with early return to sports and work. Partial weight bearing with crutches can be used in the acute phase to minimize pain and encourage a correct gait pattern, encouraging normal heel strike, protected load phase and push off (Kerkhiffs *et al.* 2001). In severe cases, early use of functional ankle supports may improve recovery times and reduced functional instability (Postle *et al.* 2012, Lin *et al.* 2010).
- Early exercises: the addition of progressive early exercises aims to restore range of motion, initiate recovery of strength and proprioception, serves to improve ankle function and aims to reduce recurrence of ankle sprains in the long term (Van Rijn *et al.* 2009, Holme *et al.* 1999).
- Cryotherapy: repeated, intermittent applications of ice to reduce pain, preferably by immersion used beyond the acute phase of ankle injury, are recommended (Bleakley *et al.* 2006, 2010).

Progressive loading/sensorimotor training phase of rehabilitation

This is the post-acute injury phase where functional and mechanical instability, chronic ankle pain and intermittent swelling are encountered.

- Manual therapy: this includes the use of active and passive joint mobilization to improve range of movement. It is essential to try to restore full dorsiflexion in weight bearing to allow a normal gait pattern and full functional recovery (Postle *et al.* 2012).
- Therapeutic exercise and activities: weight-bearing functional exercises to improve strength in the dynamic stabilizers of the ankle take several weeks. Motor coordination and balance are addressed through proprioception training, focusing on anticipation and feed-forward responses, muscle reaction timing and position/balance correction. Further evidence to determine the optimal propcioceptive training is required; however, the exercise should be made functional and relevant to individual patient demands (Postle *et al.* 2012).

Further reading

Anderson S. Evaluation and treatment of ankle sprains. *Comp Ther* 1996;**22**:30–38.

Bachmann LM, Kolb E, Koller MT, Steurer J. Accuracy of Ottawa ankle rules to exclude fractures of the ankle and mid-foot: systematic review. *Br Med J* 2003;**326(7386)**:417.

Bleakley CM, McDonough SM, MacAuley DC, Bjordal J. Cryotherapy for acute ankle sprains: a randomised controlled study of two different icing protocols. *Br J Sports Med* 2006;**40**:700–705.

Bleakley CM, O'Connor SR, Tully MA *et al.* Effect of accelerated rehabilitation on function after ankle sprain: randomised controlled trial. *Br Med J* 2010;**340**:c1964.

Chande VT. Decision rules for roentgenography of children with acute ankle injuries. *Ann Emerg Med* 1992;**21**:384–390.

Clanton TO, Porter DA. Primary care of foot and ankle injuries in the athlete. *Clin Sports Med* 1997;**16**:435.

Clark KD, Tanner S. Evaluation of the Ottawa ankle rules in children. *Ped Emerg Care* 2003;**19(2)**:73–78.

De Bie RA, de Vet HC, van den Wildenberg FA *et al.* The prognosis of ankle sprains. *Int J Sports Med* 1997;**18**:285–289.

Garrick JG, Requa RK. The epidemiology of foot and ankle injuries in sports. *Clin Sports Med* 1988;**7**(**1**):29–36.

Hattam P, Smeatham A. *Special tests in musculoskeletal examination: an evidence-based guide for clinicians*. Churchill Livingstone, London, 2010.

Holme E, Magnusson SP, Becher K *et al.* The effect of supervised rehabilitation on strength, postural sway, position sense and reinjury risk after acute ankle ligament sprain. *Scand J Med Sci Sports* 1999;**9**:104–109.

Kerkhiffs GM, Rowe BH, Assendelft WJ *et al.* Immobilisation for acute ankle sprain. A systematic review. *Arch Orthop Trauma Surg* 2001;**121**:462–471.

Lamb SE, Marsh JL, Hutton JL *et al.* Mechanical supports for acute, severe ankle sprain: a pragmatic, multicentre, randomised controlled trial. *Lancet* 2009;**373**(**9663**):575–581.

Lin C, Hiller C, de Bie R. Evidence based treatment for ankle injuries: a clinical perspective. *J Manip Ther* 2010;**18**(**1**):22–28.

Malliaropoulos N, Papacostas E, Papalada A, Maffulli N. Acute lateral ankle sprains in track and field athletes: an expanded classification. *Foot Ankle Clin* 2006;**11**:497–507.

Marder R. Current methods for the evaluation of ankle ligament injuries. *Instr Course Lect* 1995;**44**:349–357.

Matharu GC, Najran PS, Porter KM. Soft tissue ankle injuries. *Trauma* 2010;**12**:105–115.

McConnochie KM, Roghmann KJ, Pasternach J *et al.* Prediction rules for selective radiographic assessment of extremity injuries in children and adolescents. *Pediatrics* 1990;**86**:45–47.

Plint AL, Blake B, Osmond MH. Validation of the Ottawa ankle rules in children with ankle injuries. *Acad Emerg Med* 1999;**6**:1005–1009.

Postle K, Pak D, Smith TO. Effectiveness of proprioceptive exercises for ankle ligament injury in adults: a systematic literature and meta-analysis. *Man Ther* 2012;**17**(**4**):285–291.

Rubin A, Sallis R. Evaluation and diagnosis of ankle injuries. *Am Fam Phys* 1996;**54**:1609–1616.

Simon S. Structure and function of the foot and ankle. In *Orthopaedic basic science*. American Academy of Orthopaedic Surgery, Rosemont, IL, 1994, pp. 592–622.

Stiell IG, Greenberg GH, McKnight RD *et al.* A study to develop clinical decision rules for the use of radiography in acute ankle injuries. *Ann Emerg Med* 1992;**21**:384–390.

Stiell IG, Greenberg GH, McKnight RD *et al.* Decisions rules for the use of radiography in acute ankle injuries. Refinement and prospective validation. *J Am Med Assoc* 1993;**269**(**9**):1127–1132.

Tintinalli JE, Stapczynski JS, Ma OJ et al., eds. *Tintinalli's Emergency medicine: a comprehensive study guide*, 7th edn. McGraw-Hill Medical, New York, 2010.

Van Rijn RM, Van Heest JA, van der Wees P *et al.* Some benefit from physiotherapy intervention in the subgroup of patients with severe ankle sprain as determined by the ankle function score: a randomised trial. *Aust J Physiother* 2009;**55**:107–113.

Wolfe MW, Uhl TL, Mattacola CG. Management of ankle sprains. *Am Fam Physician* 2001;**63**(**1**):93–104.

CHAPTER 14

The Foot

Sherif Hemaya and Carolyn Chadwick

Sheffield Teaching Hospitals NHS Foundation Trust, Sheffield, UK

OVERVIEW

- Soft tissue problems of the foot are a common presentation and of clinical significance as they invariably result in difficulty weight bearing and mobilizing, which clearly has a significant impact upon daily life.
- This chapter addresses soft tissue pathologies of the foot commonly encountered in daily clinical practice.
- Each presentation is described according to epidemiology, clinical features and standard treatment options with a list of differential diagnoses to aid the assessing clinician.
- Additional keynotes are provided to further highlight essential clinical knowledge.

Plantar fasciitis

Introduction

This condition occurs due to inflammation and degeneration of the plantar fascia at its insertion on the medial process of the calcaneal tuberosity. The plantar fascia acts as a windlass mechanism preventing collapse of the arch of the foot while allowing shock absorption on weight bearing. Plantar fasciitis is thought to result from microtears in the fascia due to repeated biomechanical stress on the arch of the foot on weight bearing.

Epidemiology

Plantar fasciitis is the most common cause of heel pain in the adult population with an incidence of around 10%. It affects adults across the age spectrum with an incidence in women twice that of men. Ethnicity has no influence upon incidence. There is a higher preponderance in those who play sport either recreationally or professionally. Increased body weight and an increased body mass index (BMI) have also been shown to be significant risk factors for developing plantar fasciitis. Pregnancy, flat feet, high arched feet, poorly fitting or worn footwear, gait abnormalities, prolonged standing, running, jumping and walking are additional contributory factors.

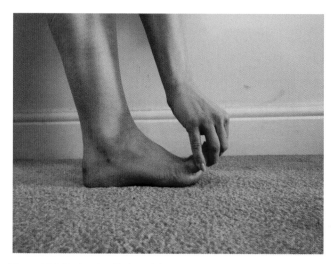

Figure 14.1 Passive dorsiflexion of the toes.

Clinical features

The patient presents with a history of severe plantar medial heel pain typically on initial mobilization after a period of non-weight bearing such as in the morning after getting up from bed or sitting for long periods. With further mobilization the pain often improves but then reoccurs and increases throughout the day with ongoing weight bearing. The diagnosis is usually made clinically with tenderness on palpation of the plantar fascia and pain on passive dorsiflexion of the toes (Figure 14.1).

Differential diagnoses

Rupture of the plantar fascia, calcaneal stress fractures (this is usually a cause of posterior heel pain), referred pain from the lumbosacral spine, disorders of the heel fat pad, ischaemic pain, tendinopathy (usually flexor hallucis longus) and tarsal tunnel syndrome (compression of the tibial nerve and its branches at the flexor retinaculum level of the ankle or in the foot) should all be considered in the differential diagnosis.

Note: ischaemic foot pain must always be considered as an important differential not to be missed. Patients may contribute presumed trauma as a suggested cause of such symptoms. It is therefore essential that a full neurovascular examination is performed on every such patient.

ABC of Common Soft Tissue Disorders, First Edition.
Edited by Francis Morris, Jim Wardrope and Paul Hattam.
© 2016 John Wiley & Sons, Ltd. Published 2016 by John Wiley & Sons, Ltd.

Treatment

The condition is typically self-limiting with spontaneous resolution in more than 90% of cases by 1 year. Traditional treatment regimens are predominantly non-operative. They involve patient education, ensuring correct footwear and anti-inflammatory drugs (both systemic and topical) with adequate analgesia. Rest and modification of daily activities in relation to weight bearing also need to be addressed along with other physical therapies.

The initial therapy employed is icing, by either rubbing/massaging an ice cube or ice pack directly onto the heel and sole of the foot or by soaking the heel and plantar aspect of the foot in an ice bath, taking care to avoid cold injury.

The second aspect of physical therapy is stretching exercises of the plantar fascia, calf muscles and Achilles tendon. Stretching of the plantar fascia is achieved by deep massage of the fascia with the toes dorsiflexed (Figure 14.2). Rolling a can (ideally frozen to provide the additional benefit of icing) or golf ball with the foot also allows stretching of the fascia (Figure 14.3). Toe curls can also be performed to strengthen foot musculature (Figure 14.4).

Calf and Achilles stretching is achieved by performing asymmetrical stretching exercises (Figure 14.5).

Cushioned heel inserts and night splints may also be beneficial. If this approach fails further therapies are corticosteroid injection and newer treatment options such as platelet-rich plasma (PRP) injection and extracorporeal shockwave therapy. Rarely surgery is carried out in cases resistant to at least 12 months of conservative measures.

Metatarsalgia

Introduction

A term describing pain from any cause underneath the metatarsal heads, this commonly occurs as a result of increased stress on the plantar region of the forefoot.

Epidemiology

Participants in high-impact sports that place considerable transfer of force to the forefoot are commonly affected.

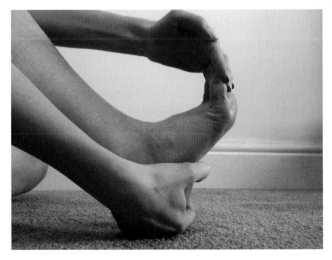

Figure 14.2 Rubbing the plantar fascia with toes dorsiflexed.

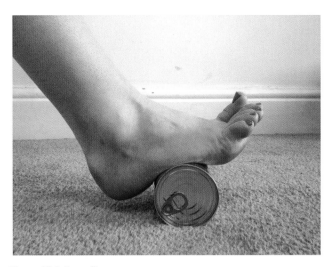

Figure 14.3 Can rolling.

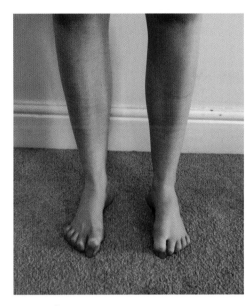

Figure 14.4 Toe curling.

Clinical features

There is pain at one or more of the metatarsal heads of gradual rather than sudden onset, unless due to an acute injury such as plantar plate rupture or fracture. The metatarsal squeeze test is useful for eliciting symptoms.

Differential diagnoses

Stress fracture, inflammatory arthropathy (such as gout), bursitis, plantar plate rupture, fat pad atrophy, interdigital neuroma and lesser toe deformities.

Treatment

Treatment is conservative, including footwear modification such as avoiding high heels. In addition, orthotics are used to redistribute pressure under the foot and offload the metatarsal heads such as a metatarsal bar. Achilles tendon stretching is indicated if contracted

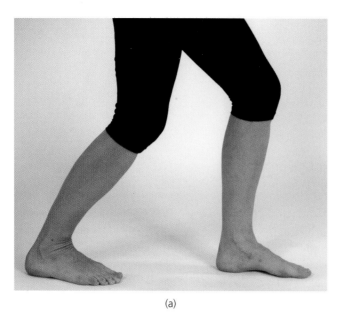 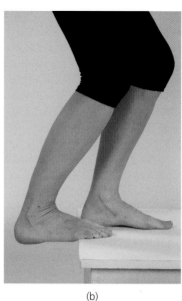

(a)   (b)

Figure 14.5 Calf stretch. (a) Flat on the floor; (b) on a step.

and weight loss is necessary in those who are overweight. Surgery may be indicated if conservative measures fail depending on the underlying diagnosis.

Pearls and pitfalls

A Morton's (interdigital) neuroma causes irritation and inflammation of the digital nerve in the web space between the metatarsal heads. This mechanical entrapment neuropathy therefore produces prominent metatarsalgia symptoms. Such symptoms will often include burning, numbness and tingling to the toes in addition to pain. Symptoms may be worsened on lateral foot/metatarsal squeeze.

Extensor tendinopathy

Introduction

Extensor tendinopathy produces pain across the dorsum of the foot. It is typically caused by inadequate footwear, which leads to direct pressure on these tendons resulting in inflammation, and subsequently pain and swelling.

Epidemiology

More commonly affected is the extensor hallucis longus and adults of all ages are affected, particularly those who weight bear for long periods including walking and running, especially in tightly fitting shoes. Direct trauma can also occur in addition to kicking injuries. Other risk factors for developing the condition are high arched feet and flat feet.

Clinical features

Patients will complain of pain to the dorsum of the foot that is worsened by movement and relieved with rest. Dorsal foot tenderness, swelling and occasionally bruising may be evident. Resisted extension of the toes causes pain.

Differential diagnoses

Gout, metatarsal fracture, degenerative arthropathy and complex regional pain syndrome (CRPS; see below).

Treatment

The mainstay of treatment involves patient education, change to comfortable, loose-fitting footwear, modification of daily activities, calf muscle stretching, ice, anti-inflammatory drugs (both topical and systemic) and analgesia. Additional treatment modalities are ultrasound therapy, orthotic insoles and shoe inserts as well as local steroid injection into the affected tendon sheath. This is, however, associated with the risk of tendon rupture. Severe cases may require a removable below-knee cast/splint.

Pearls and pitfalls

Always consider the possibility of a metatarsal stress fracture in patients presenting with pain and swelling isolated to the second or third metatarsals.

Tibialis posterior tendinopathy

Introduction

This is more commonly an intrinsic abnormality within the tendon or biomechanical failure due to chronic repetitive stress. It may also occur following an acute traumatic injury. Medial ankle sprains sustained with the foot pronated and everted can result in tenosynovitis with subsequent degeneration and stretching of the tendon, contributing to a flat foot deformity that worsens progressively over years. If untreated the tibialis posterior tendon may eventually rupture. Acute ruptures of the tendon are rare.

Epidemiology

Women are more commonly affected than men, with a typical age older than 40 years. Obesity and diabetes are additional risk factors. High-impact sports are a risk factor in younger patients.

Clinical features

There is typically persistent medial ankle pain, with or without swelling, to the medial aspect of the ankle following a minor injury or sprain, worsened by activity. In the early stages the medial arch of the foot is maintained. In later stages of disease progression the heel tilts outward and a flat foot deformity is present. Standing behind the patient the 'too many toes' sign will be evident. The patient will also be unable to perform the single-limb heel rise test, which involves standing on one leg on tip toes (Figure 14.6).

Differential diagnoses

This condition is commonly misdiagnosed as a medial ankle sprain in the absence of a history of acute trauma. When in doubt musculoskeletal ultrasound or magnetic resonance imaging (MRI) will confirm the diagnosis.

Treatment

Conservative measures are instituted initially including analgesia, non-steroidal anti-inflammatory drugs (NSAIDs), patient education, activity modification and rest to offload the tendon with the use of a short leg cast, removable walking boots (Figure 14.7) or an orthotic. Surgical treatment is reserved for those with no improvement following a minimum 6 months of conservative treatment.

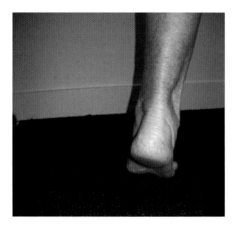

Figure 14.6 The single-limb heel rise test.

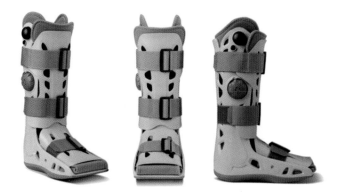

Figure 14.7 Walking boot.

Pearls and pitfalls

The diagnosis of a medial ankle sprain should not be made in the absence of a history of direct acute trauma due to the particularly debilitating and potentially progressive nature of tibialis posterior tendinopathy. Appropriate follow-up is advised for such patients.

Stress fracture

Introduction

Stress fractures are common and are caused by repeated and recurrent loading on the bone resulting in bone fatigue and eventual fracture. Typical sites in the foot are the second metatarsal shaft but other metatarsals can also be affected as well as the navicular.

Epidemiology

Prolonged or unusual exercise is the typical cause, often with an increase or change to activity level. There is seldom a history of trauma preceding symptoms and therefore there is a tendency to label them as soft tissue 'sprains'. Additional risk factors are osteoporosis, menstrual disturbance in young females, dietary restriction and rheumatoid disease.

Clinical features

There will be swelling to the dorsal aspect of the foot with localized bony tenderness to the navicular or metatarsal shafts. Initial x-rays are often normal with periosteal reaction appearing after 2–4 weeks. A bone scan may be required to make a formal diagnosis.

Differential diagnoses

Extensor tendinopathy, metatarsalgia and interdigital neuroma.

Treatment

Symptomatic relief with reduction of activity, rest, elevation, ice, analgesia and wearing comfortable, firm-fitting footwear with good padding to the insole. In patients unable to weight bear a below-knee plaster cast may be required with the use of crutches or a removable walking boot (Figure 14.7). Recovery should take around 6–8 weeks.

Complex regional pain syndrome (CRPS)

Introduction

There are two categories of CRPS. CRPS I, also known as reflex sympathetic dystrophy, is a non-specific pain syndrome following trauma. CRPS II results from direct injury to a nerve.

Epidemiology

Women are more commonly affected by this condition with a peak incidence in those aged 20–35 years. Children can also be affected although it is rare under the age of 10 years. There is a strong association with cigarette smoking. The pathophysiology is complex, involving all parts of the neurological system.

Clinical features

The main symptom of CRPS I is chronic worsening of spontaneous, severe pain disproportionate to the initial trauma sustained. The pain does not typically follow a single nerve distribution and is worsened by movement of the affected limb with muscle fatigability. There is difficulty experienced in using the affected limb and the patient often demonstrates symptoms of neglect, either motor or cognitive. Muscle spasms, tremor and dystonia may occur and there is commonly disuse atrophy.

Sensory disturbance is often present, with allodynia (pain on touch) and hypoaesthesia (reduced sensation). This often follows a glove-and-stocking distribution and may be heightened while pain is being experienced as well as an exaggerated response to painful stimulus.

Vasomotor disturbance manifests as a difference in skin temperature between affected and unaffected limbs as well as skin colour changes, with the skin appearing shiny, dry or scaly. Hair may be initially coarse before becoming thin, and nail growth is impaired. Autonomic disturbance is demonstrated by abnormal sweating and limb oedema.

Treatment

Treatment should be multidisciplinary (anaesthetist, psychologist, orthopaedic surgeon, neurologist, physiotherapist), with NSAIDs, physiotherapy and occupational therapy, as well as other therapies aimed at helping a patient with chronic pain. Nerve block, epidural injection, dorsal column stimulator and surgical sympathectomy have been utilized with varying success.

Pearls and pitfalls

Consider CRPS in those patients with a disproportionate amount of pain from an injury with autonomic limb signs and symptoms with no other explainable pathology. Early diagnosis and aggressive management to maintain range of movement give a better prognosis.

Further reading

Bulstrode C, Wilson-Macdonald J, Eastwood D *et al. Oxford textbook of trauma and orthopaedics.* Oxford University Press, Oxford, 2011.

Marx J, Hockberger R, Walls R. *Rosen's emergency medicine - concepts and clinical practice.* Elsevier Saunders Publishing, Philadelphia, PA, 2014.

Medscape online resourceshttp://emedicine.medscape.com

Patient.co.uk online resourceshttp://www.patient.co.uk

Index

ABC of Common Soft Tissue Disorders, First Edition.
Edited by Francis Morris, Jim Wardrope and Paul Hattam.
© 2016 John Wiley & Sons, Ltd. Published 2016 by John Wiley & Sons, Ltd.